Essential Notes on Prescribing for Finals and Junior Doctors

RAHIL D MANDALIA
MBBS BSc (Hons)
Foundation Doctor
University Hospitals of Leicester

and

KARTIK LOGISHETTY
MBBS BSc (Hons)
Academic Foundation Doctor
Oxford University Hospitals

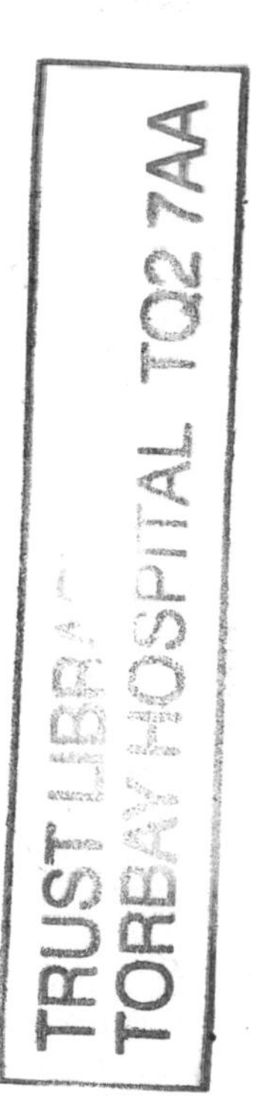

Foreword by

THOMPSON ROBINSON
BMedSci MD FRCP
Professor of Stroke Medicine
University Hospitals of Leicester

Radcliffe Publishing
London • New York

Radcliffe Publishing Ltd
33–41 Dallington Street
London
EC1V 0BB
United Kingdom

www.radcliffepublishing.com

Every effort has been made to ensure that the information in this book is accurate. This does not diminish the requirement to exercise clinical judgement, and neither the publisher nor the authors can accept any responsibility for its use in practice.

New research and clinical experience can result in changes in treatment and drug therapy. Users of the information in this book should therefore check the most recent product information on any drug they may prescribe to ensure they are complying with the manufacturer's recommendations concerning dosage, the method and duration of administration and contraindications.

British Library Cataloguing in Publication Data

A catalogue record for this book is available from the British Library.

ISBN-13: 978 184619 967 7

The paper used for the text pages of this book is FSC® certified. FSC (The Forest Stewardship Council®) is an international network to promote responsible management of the world's forests.

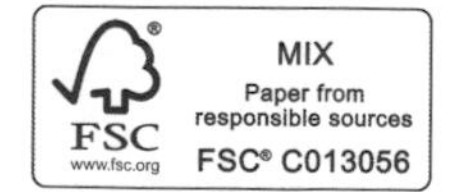

Typeset by Darkriver Design, Auckland, New Zealand
Printed and bound by TJI Digital, Padstow, Cornwall, UK

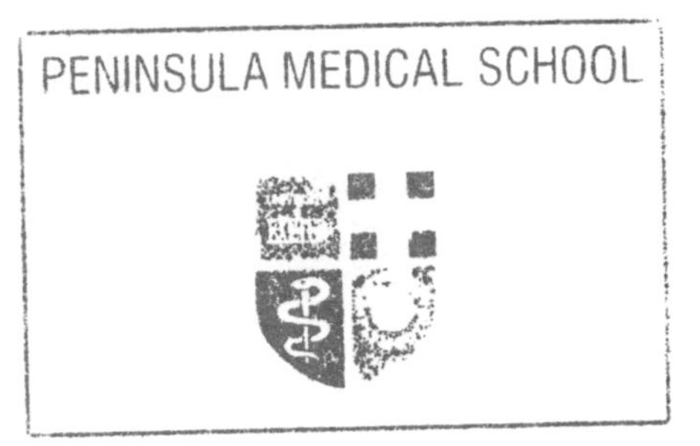

Contents

Foreword

In this book, *Essential Notes on Prescribing for Finals and Junior Doctors*, Drs Rahil Mandalia and Kartik Logishetty provide important advice on prescribing, together with practical examples of prescribing in common conditions. The ability to prescribe is an important duty of a doctor; the General Medical Council clearly defines 'the ability to prescribe drugs, with adequate knowledge of the patient's health, and satisfied that the drugs serve the patient's needs' as an important principle of providing good clinical care within the principles of Good Medical Practice. Furthermore, research commissioned by the General Medical Council has identified an error rate of 8.9% in hospital prescriptions, many written by foundation doctors. Therefore, this book will not just be helpful in preparation for final clinical and written examinations, but also in your early career as a foundation doctor.

Thompson Robinson BMedSci MD FRCP
Professor of Stroke Medicine
University Hospitals of Leicester
June 2012

Preface

This text aims to provide the senior medical student and the foundation doctor with the knowledge and confidence to prescribe safely and appropriately.

We begin by introducing the standard prescription chart, and discussing key considerations, dangers and pitfalls. This simple framework offers a base for the rest of the text.

The initial chapters approach regularly encountered problems seen on the hospital ward and reflect clinical practice. While the undergraduate medical curriculum teaches the pharmacological and therapeutic aspects of commonly used medications, this text addresses the transition between learning medicine and practising it.

Chapter 10 provides a number of prescribing challenges often presented in medical school examinations and offers a useful reference for the foundation doctor. These are presented as clinical vignettes, with corresponding drug treatments written as prescription charts.

Prescribing is a prerequisite skill of all medical graduates. It is notoriously difficult to teach and develop, relying on a thorough foundation of knowledge and practical application. Here we offer a step-by-step guide to prescribing as a platform for the junior doctor.

Rahil D Mandalia
Kartik Logishetty
June 2012

1

Practical prescribing

Prescription charts are composed of the following sections:

1. a. Patient details
   b. Allergies and sensitivities
2. Once-only medications
3. Regular medications
4. As-required medications
5. Oxygen prescriptions
6. Complex and variable dose medications:
   a. anticoagulation
   b. patient-controlled analgesia
7. Infusion therapy/fluids

1a. Patient details; 1b. Allergies and sensitivities

INPATIENT PRESCRIPTION CHART

ALLERGIES & SENSITIVITY (Use red ink & give details)		
Hospital:	Weight (kg)	Height (m)
Ward:	Diet	Tick if active oncology chart
Consultant:		☐

Hospital No:	D.O.B:
Surname:	
First Name:	
Address:	
	Sex: M / F
OR USE PATIENT LABEL	

2. Once-only medications

ONCE ONLY & PRE-ANAESTHETIC MEDICATION

PRESCRIBED		DRUG	ROUTE	DOSE	PRESCRIBER'S SIGNATURE	GIVEN BY	TIME GIVEN	PHARMACY
DATE	TIME	(approved name)						

3. Regular medications

REGULAR PRESCRIPTIONS NAME: Hosp. No:

YEAR:	**MONTH:**		**DATE →**			
			Time ↓	**Week 1**	**Week 2**	**Week 3**
DRUG (approved name)			0600			
DOSE	ROUTE	Pharmacy	0800			
Instructions/Duration			1300			
Start Date & Time			1800			
Signature			2200			
CANCEL (Date & Sig)			0000			
DRUG (approved name)			0600			
DOSE	ROUTE	Pharmacy	0800			
Instructions/Duration			1300			
Start Date & Time			1800			
Signature			2200			
CANCEL (Date & Sig)			0000			
DRUG (approved name)			0600			

4. As-required medications

AS REQUIRED PRESCRIPTIONS NAME: Hosp. No:

DRUG (approved name)		ROUTE	I	C	**Date**	
DOSE & Maximum Frequency		PHARMACY			**Time**	
					Dose	
Start Date & Time	TTAs	CANCEL (Date & Sig)			**Route**	
Signature					**Given By**	
DRUG (approved name)		ROUTE	I	C	**Date**	
DOSE & Maximum Frequency		PHARMACY			**Time**	
					Dose	
Start Date & Time	TTAs	CANCEL (Date & Sig)			**Route**	
Signature					**Given By**	

5. Oxygen prescriptions

OXYGEN PRESCRIPTIONS NAME: Hosp. No:

OXYGEN REGIME TARGETS							
TARGET OXYGEN SATURATION							
88–92%	☐	94–98%	☐	OTHER			
CONTINUOUS	☐	PRN	☐	———			
MAX OXYGEN %							
21	24	28	35	40	60	80	98
MAX FLOW RATE L/min							
2	4	6	8	10	12	15	High flow >15 L/min
DATE							
TIME							
SIGNATURE							
CANCEL (Date & Sig)							

DATE	TIME	DEVICE	SpO2	OXYGEN %	FLOW RATE	Administrator SIGNATURE

OXYGEN REGIME TARGETS							
TARGET OXYGEN SATURATION							
88–92%	☐	94–98%	☐	OTHER			
CONTINUOUS	☐	PRN	☐	———			
MAX OXYGEN %							
21	24	28	35	40	60	80	98
MAX FLOW RATE L/min							
2	4	6	8	10	12	15	High flow >15 L/min
DATE							
TIME							
SIGNATURE							
CANCEL (Date & Sig)							

DATE	TIME	DEVICE	SpO2	OXYGEN %	FLOW RATE	Administrator SIGNATURE

6. Complex and variable dose medications

COMPLEX & VARIABLE DOSE PRESCRIPTIONS NAME: Hosp. No:

DRUG (approved name)	
DOSE & INSTRUCTIONS **(Specify monitoring variables, frequency or any protocol)**	
ROUTE	**PHARMACY**
Start Date & Time	
Sig.	**CANCEL** **(Date & Sig)**

Date	Time	Observation	Dose	Signature	Given By

7. Infusion therapy/fluids

INFUSION THERAPY PATIENT'S NAME: Hosp. No:

DATE	FLUID	VOL	RATE	ROUTE	BATCH NO.	DRUG ADDED	DOSE	DOCTOR'S SIGNATURE	DATE & TIME		SET UP BY	CHECKED BY
									BEGUN	ENDED		

1a. Patient details

- Verbally check the patient's name and details.
- Use electronic labels where possible.

1b. Allergies and sensitivities

- Verbally check these with the patient, and do not rely on previous notes.
- Document allergies or sensitivities in red ink on the chart, and it is good practice to document the nature of the associated reaction.
- Note that all unexpected adverse reactions should be investigated and reported by the yellow card system.

Medications

- Drugs should be prescribed by their generic name.
- Decimal points should be avoided where possible.
- Quantities less than 1 gram should be written in milligrams, and quantities less than 1 milligram should be written in micrograms.
- 'Micrograms', 'nanograms' and 'units' should not be abbreviated.

All drug prescriptions should be written in capital letters and black ink, and as a minimum should contain the following:

Drug Name I Dose (units) I Route of Administration I Date of Prescription I Name of Prescriber I Signature I Contact Details

ABBREVIATION	TRANSLATION
o.d. (omni die)	Once a day
b.d. or b.i.d. (bis die)	Twice a day
t.d.s. or t.i.d. (ter die sumendus)	Three times a day
q.d.s. (quarter die sumendus)	Four times a day
p.o. (per os)	Oral route
p.r. (per rectum)	Rectal route
p.v. (per vaginum)	Vaginal route
s.c.	Subcutaneous
i.m.	Intramuscular
i.v.	Intravenous
s.l.	Sublingual
top.	Topical
mane	In the morning
nocte	At night
p.r.n. (pro re nata)	As required
stat. (statim)	Immediately
T, TT, TTT or i, ii, iii	One, Two, Three (tablets)

2. Once-only or single-dose medication

- These are often drugs given in emergencies.
- In addition to the above, document the time at which the drug is to be administered.

3. Regular medications

- Always document the times at which the medication should be given.
- For medication given more than once a day, space intervals evenly.
- Where appropriate, for example when prescribing antibiotics, document the indication for the drug and an end date for the prescription.

4. As-required medications ('p.r.n.')

- Always document the minimum dose interval.
- This can be documented by a maximum frequency (e.g. every 4 hours) or by a maximum dose (e.g. total 1 g every day).

5. Oxygen prescriptions

- As a minimum, prescriptions for oxygen require the following:

Date | Device | Oxygen % | Flow Rate (L/min) | Target Oxygen Saturation | Prescriber Name | Signature | Contact Details |

- Two separate oxygen prescriptions may be required, to denote continuous and p.r.n. therapy.

6. Complex and variable dose medications

a. Some drug charts contain specific sections for the prescription of anticoagulants such as warfarin, where 'Target INR' must be documented.
b. There may be a section for prescription of patient-controlled analgesia.

- In addition to Drug Name, Bolus Dose, Background Infusion, and Lock-out Time, you must also prescribe a reversal agent and dose.

7. Infusion therapy/fluids

- This is often on the back of the drug prescription chart. Prescriptions of infusions require the following:

Date | Name of Fluid | Volume | Rate of Infusion | Route of Infusion | Name of Drug Added | Dose of Drug Added | Name of Prescriber | Signature | Contact Details |

- The 'Rate of Infusion' may either be written as a total time for the infusion to be completed in (e.g. over 8 hours) or as a rate (e.g. 125 mL/hr).

Controlled drugs

- Outpatient prescriptions for controlled drugs require a different format for legal requirements. The entire prescription must be handwritten in indelible ink.
- You must document the total quantity of the preparation in words AND FIGURES. For example:

Drug Name | Dose (units) | Route of administration | Date of Prescription | Name of Prescriber | Signature | Contact Details
Total quantity supplied:

Morphine Sulphate IR (Oramorph) (1 mg/mL) | 5–10 mL (Five to Ten Millilitres) | p.o. | Q.D.S. | 19/1/20 | Dr David Robbins
Total quantity supplied: 100 mL (One Hundred Millilitres)

Adverse drug reactions

> *An adverse drug reaction (ADR) is an unwanted or harmful reaction experienced following the administration of a drug or combination of drugs under normal conditions of use and is suspected to be related to the drug.*
>
> —*MHRA Yellow Card Scheme*

ADRs are responsible for up to 5% of hospital admissions and occur in up to one-fifth of hospitalised patients. Take a clear drug history of the patient, noting current and past medication. It is also important to ask about the nature and symptoms of any previous reactions, and whether any medications or doses were altered due to previous ADRs.

There are seven types of ADR, of which Type A is the commonest (up to 80%).

- **Type A *(Augmented)*:** This is due to dose-dependent *augmentation* of the drug. Reducing the dose of the drug will reduce or prevent this ADR.
  —Example: over-warfarinisation of a patient.
- **Type B *(Bizarre)*:** These are usually severe, unpredictable and not dose related, and are thought to be a consequence of human metabolism. As they are rare (about 1 in 10 000), they are less likely to be observed in clinical trials, and are often found after trials.
  —Example: penicillin anaphylaxis.
- **Type C *(Chronic treatment)*:** These are due to long-term treatment with a drug.
  —Example: immunosuppression with steroid use.
- **Type D *(Delayed effect)*:** Can occur after a period of time following termination of the drug.
  —Example: cancers due to use of immunosuppression.
- **Type E *(End of treatment)*:** Due to withdrawal of a drug.
  —Example: benzodiazepines.
- **Type F *(Failure of therapy)*:** This is a drug interaction where one drug can reduce the efficacy of another.
  —Example: St John's wort and theophylline.

- **Type G *(Genetic)*:** Are due to direct genetic damage.
  —Example: teratogenicity of thalidomide.

Prescribing for the vulnerable patient

Children

The *British National Formulary* written for paediatrics offers appropriate drug regimens for children. Dosage is often based on body surface area or weight. Liquid preparations are particularly suitable. Avoid intramuscular injections in children because they tend to be very painful.

Neonates have a more permeable blood–brain barrier than adults. They are therefore more susceptible to centrally acting drugs, and due care should be taken.

Elderly

In normal ageing there is:

- a decreased distribution of hydrosoluble drugs (due to a lower overall percentage of body water) and an increased distribution of liposoluble drugs (due to a higher proportion of fat) relative to the younger adult; liposoluble drugs can therefore accumulate
- a decreased hepatic mass and blood flow, causing reduced first-pass, and phase 1 metabolism, oxidation, reduction, and hydrolysis
- reduced renal clearance
- a reduced response to beta agonists and blockers
- an increased response to opiates, benzodiazepines and warfarin.

Once an elderly patient is taking four or more medications, there is a considerable increase in the risk of adverse drug reactions. Therefore, where possible do the following:

1. Simplify the drug schedule.
2. Reduce 'as required' medications.
3. Prescribe slow-release medications where appropriate.
4. Limit the number of medications concurrently prescribed.

Where possible, avoid the following drugs:

- Hypnotics: elderly patients are particularly susceptible to confusion, ataxia, slurred speech, and imbalance resulting in falls.
- Diuretics: electrolyte disturbances are more common. A low-volume state may manifest as postural hypotension and subsequently increase the risk of falls.
- NSAIDs: there is an increased tendency to bleed from the gastrointestinal tract, in addition to an increased risk of renal failure in the elderly.
- Antiparkinsonian drugs, antihypertensives, psychotropics and digoxin commonly cause adverse drug reactions in the elderly. A lower dose of opiates, benzodiazepines and warfarin are often required.

Pregnancy

- Avoid all drugs in the first trimester if possible. This is because there is a high risk of teratogenesis between weeks 3 and 11 of pregnancy.
- Drugs given in the second and third trimester may affect growth or have toxic effects on tissue.
- Warfarin is teratogenic. Patients who require anticoagulation and are pregnant or at risk of becoming pregnant should be prescribed heparin.
- Methotrexate can cause foetal abnormalities long after its cessation. Therefore, couples should be advised to avoid conceiving for at least 3 months after stopping methotrexate.
- Many chemotherapy agents are teratogenic.

Breast feeding

- Certain drugs have a propensity to be present in breast milk.
- Neonates have immature excretory function. Drugs consumed in breast milk may therefore accumulate and have toxic effects.
- Others such as bromocriptine can affect lactation.

- Common drugs to avoid during pregnancy include:
  - —aspirin (Reye's syndrome)
  - —captopril
  - —ciprofloxacin
  - —enoxaparin
  - —antipsychotics
  - —lithium.
- A more comprehensive list can be found in the latest *British National Formulary* (BNF).

References

Joint Formulary Committee, editors. *British National Formulary 63*. British Medical Association, Royal Pharmaceutical Society of Great Britain; 2012.

Medicines and Healthcare Products Regulatory Agency. *Yellow Card System – Reporting Adverse Drug Reactions*. Available online at: www.mhra.gov.uk/Safetyinformation/Reportingsafetyproblems/ (accessed 8 May 2012).

2

Oxygen therapy

Respiratory failure (RF) is a common condition of patients in hospital and is a consequence of inadequate gas exchange. Classification of respiratory failure is as follows.

- Type 1 RF is due to *oxygenation failure* and leads to *hypoxaemia with normo- or hypocapnia.* This is most often due to a ventilation/perfusion (V/Q) mismatch, where the lungs are adequately perfused but inadequately ventilated.

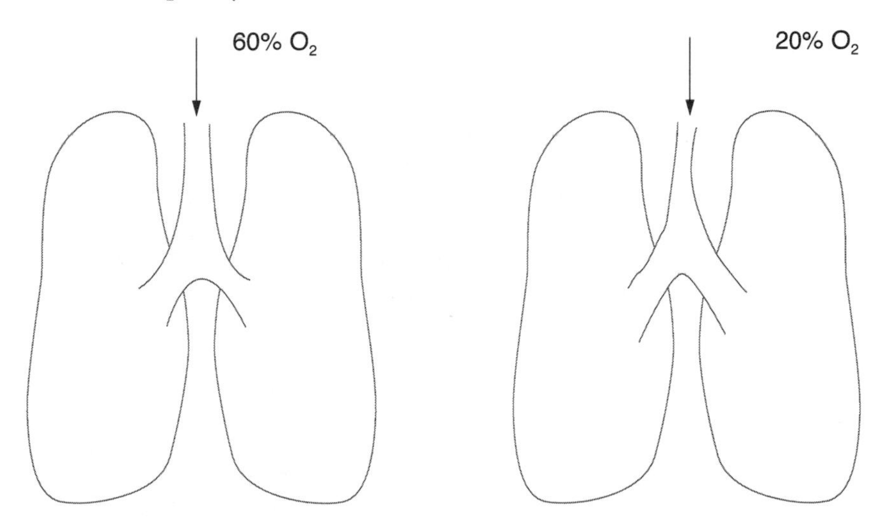

- Type 2 RF is due to *ventilatory failure* and is characterised by *hypercapnia with or without hypoxaemia*. This is due to the inability of the lungs to blow off CO_2 due to alveolar hypoventilation.

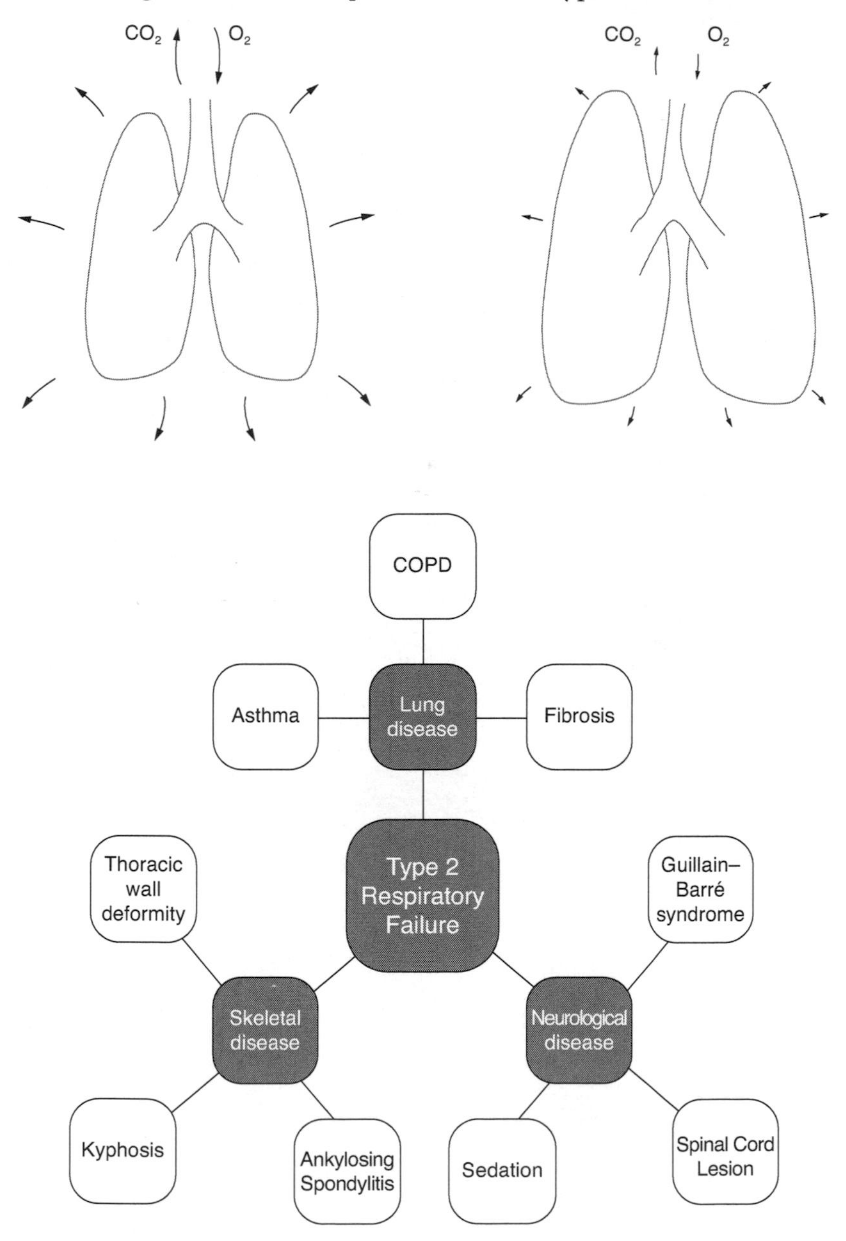

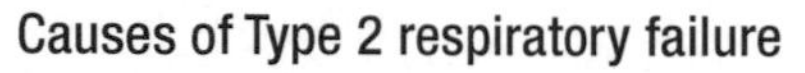

Causes of Type 2 respiratory failure

Respiratory drive is normally dependent upon arterial CO_2. Hydrogen ions released as a consequence of CO_2 hydration in brain tissue have a direct action on **central chemoreceptors** to increase the work and rate of breathing (**hypercarbic drive**).

Over time, patients with Type 2 respiratory failure may become increasingly insensitive to CO_2, and instead depend upon their **hypoxic drive** to breathe. In such patients, caution must be taken when prescribing oxygen, as prescribing too much may reduce their hypoxic drive – resulting in apnoea.

Oxygen therapy aims to alleviate respiratory failure and prevent tissue hypoxia by increasing the fraction of inspired oxygen (FiO_2) to above 21%. There are a number of ways of delivering oxygen to be aware of (*see* pages 18–23).

Simple face mask

These masks are often seen in hospital and connected to wall oxygen. They provide a *variable* delivery of oxygen as the FiO_2 depends upon patient ventilation. Hence they are avoided in patients with *ventilatory failure* (T2RF). Oxygen flows into the mask at a set rate (L/min) and air is drawn into the mask from the side of the mask at a rate dependent upon patient ventilation.

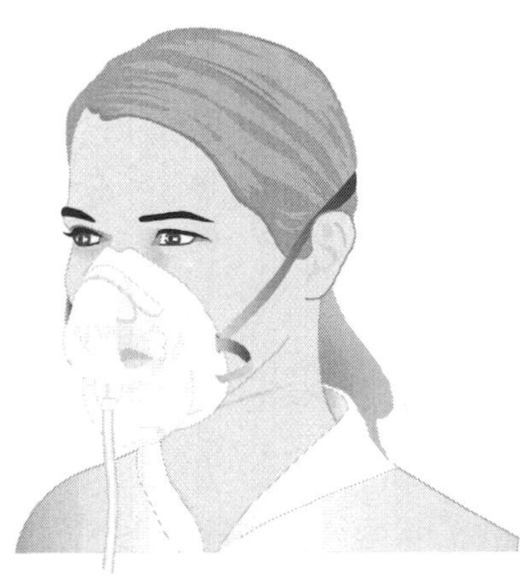

Nasal prongs

These are similar to low flow masks and work under the same principle. At flow rates of approximately 2–4 litres per minute they are comfortable and allow the patient to talk and eat during oxygen therapy. High flows are avoided, as they can be uncomfortable for the patient.

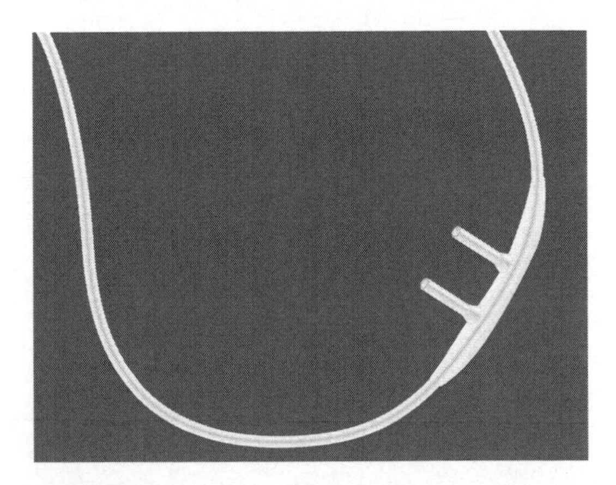

Non-rebreather mask

This is another mask that gives a *variable* delivery of oxygen as the FiO_2 depends upon patient ventilation. Overall it delivers a higher FiO_2 than low-flow masks and nasal prongs as it contains a reservoir bag and one-way valve. It is used in patients that require a high FiO_2 in an emergency. *N.B.* No mask can deliver 100% FiO_2.

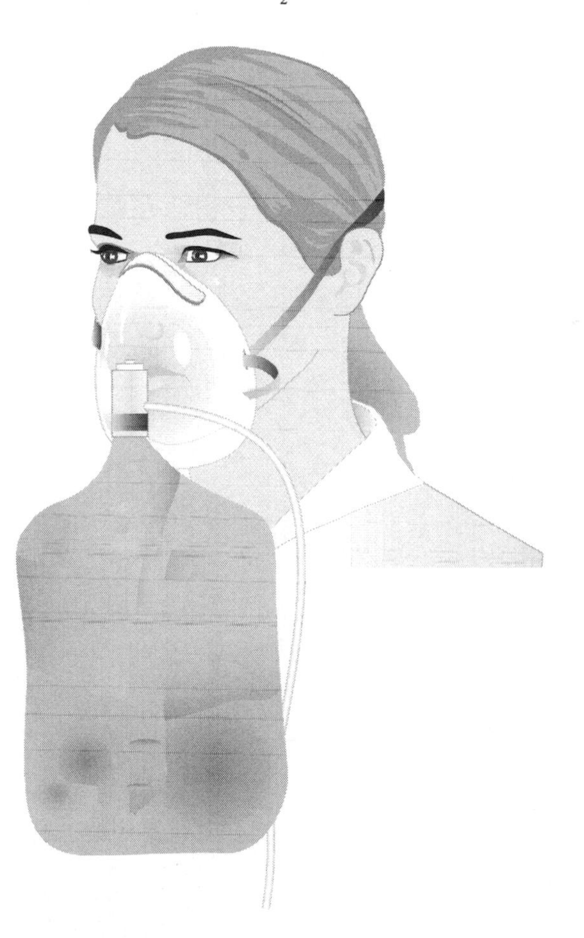

Venturi masks

These masks provide a fixed FiO_2 by the use of a Venturi adapter, which is colour coded. They allow the entrainment of room air to a fixed oxygen source from the wall outlet. This combination leads to an accurate estimation of FiO_2 and facilitates tailored oxygen therapy, which is ideal for patients who depend upon their hypoxic drive to breathe.

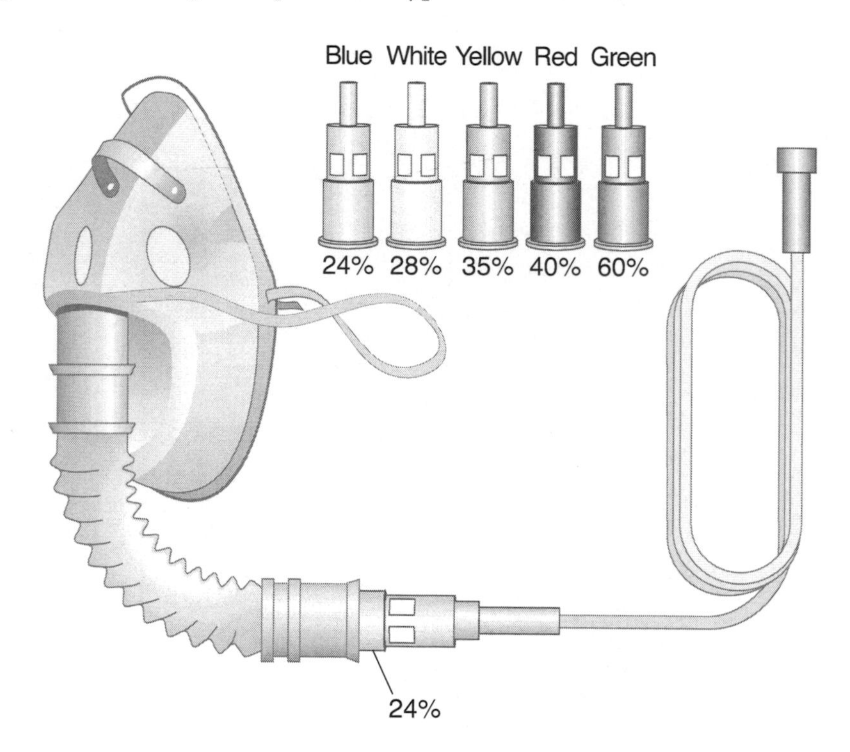

ADAPTOR COLOUR	O_2 FLOW RATE (L/MIN)	FIO_2 (%)
Blue	3	24
Yellow	6	28
White	8	31
Green	12	35
Pink	15	40
Orange	15	50

Non-invasive ventilation

In the conscious, tolerating patient who remains hypoxaemic despite the above interventions, consider non-invasive ventilation (NIV).

1. Continuous positive airways pressure (CPAP)

CPAP provides a continuous pressure of 5–10 cmH_2O through both inspiration and expiration. This prevents alveolar collapse during the respiratory cycle, thereby increasing oxygenation.

Uses:

- obstructive sleep apnoea
- cardiogenic pulmonary oedema
- pneumonia
- exacerbation of COPD.

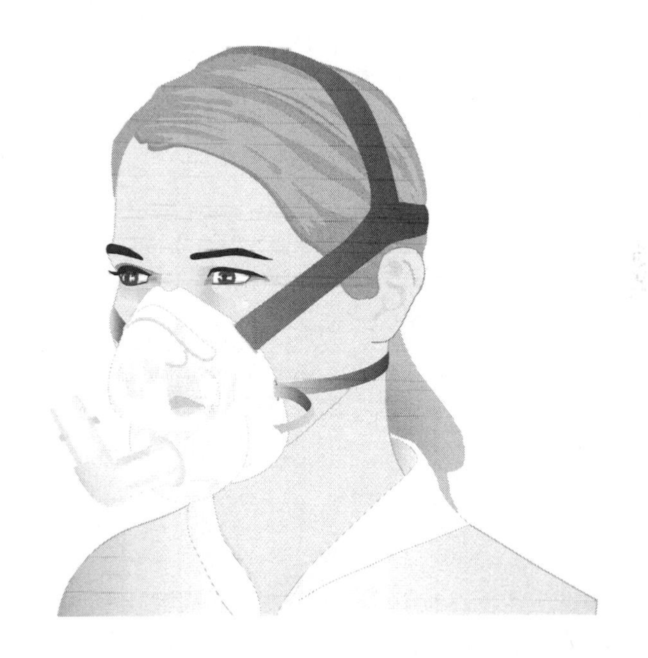

2. Bilevel positive airway pressure (BiPAP)

BiPAP is used to provide adequate non-invasive ventilatory support for hypercapnic respiratory failure. It delivers two levels of pressure (inspiratory positive airway pressure (IPAP) and expiratory positive airway pressure (EPAP). The IPAP augments ventilation and the EPAP prevents alveolar collapse (like CPAP).

Uses:

- exacerbations of COPD with T2RF
- neuromuscular disease
- chest wall deformity
- obstructive sleep apnoea with T2RF.

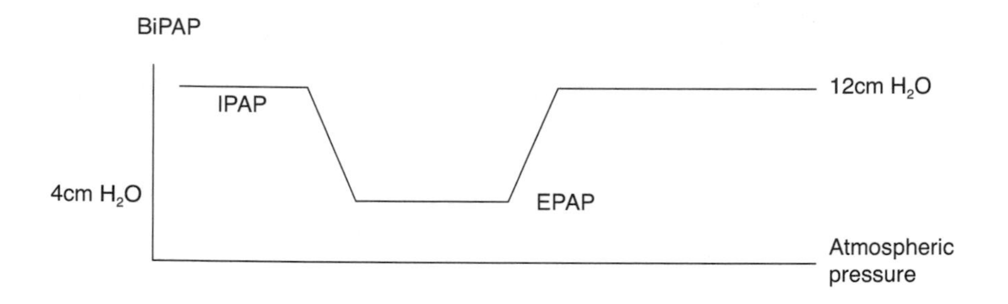

Invasive ventilation

Tracheal intubation may be indicated in patients that are deteriorating due to:

- respiratory failure (hypoxaemia, hypercapnia, respiratory acidosis)
- upper airway obstruction, e.g. laryngospasm, inhalation burn, epiglottitis
- major haemodynamic instability requiring inotropic support
- reduced consciousness with loss of gag reflex (GCS of 8 or below).

References

British Thoracic Society Standards of Care Committee. Non-invasive ventilation in acute respiratory failure. *Thorax*. 2002; **57**(3): 192–211.

O'Driscoll BR, Howard LS, Davison AG. BTS guideline for emergency oxygen use in adult patients. *Thorax*. 2008; **63**(Suppl VI): vi1–vi68.

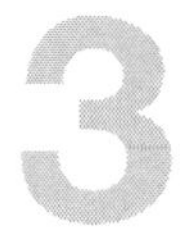

Analgesia and palliative care

Analgesia

Before prescribing analgesia, take a good history and treat the underlying cause of pain wherever possible. Once prescribed, patients with pain must be reviewed regularly. Oral analgesia should be tried before the parenteral route where possible.

WHO analgesic ladder

STEP 1
Paracetamol and/or NSAID (plus adjuvant)

STEP 2
Paracetamol and/or NSAID
ADD weak opioid for mild/moderate pain (plus adjuvant)

STEP 3
Paracetamol and/or NSAID
ADD strong opioid for severe pain (plus adjuvant)

Note that any combination of NSAID with aspirin, corticosteroid, and/or anticoagulant will increase the risk of gastrointestinal toxicity. A proton-pump inhibitor should be co-prescribed.

Analgesics

Paracetamol

Mechanism of action: It is an antipyretic and analgesic, but has no anti-inflammatory properties. It works by inhibiting cyclo-oxygenase (COX), which results in a reduction in the formation of prostaglandins from arachidonic acid.

Indications: Mild to moderate pain, pyrexia.

Contraindications and cautions: Beware of dose-related toxicity, particularly in those with hepatic impairment.

Dose: Paracetamol, 500 mg–1 g q.d.s. p.o./i.v., max 4 g daily.

Non-steroidal anti-inflammatory drugs (NSAIDs)

Mechanism of action: These are cyclo-oxygenase (COX) inhibitors. COX exists in two isoforms, COX-1 and COX-2. It is the inhibition of COX-1 that is thought to be responsible for gastric ulceration related to NSAID use. Selective COX-2 inhibitors are associated with less gastrointestinal intolerance, though there are concerns surrounding their cardiovascular safety.

Indications: Continuous or regular pain associated with inflammation, back pain, soft-tissue disorders.

Examples: Ibuprofen, naproxen, diclofenac, celecoxib (a selective COX-2 inhibitor).

Contraindications and cautions: Caution in elderly, contraindicated in patients with history of hypersensitivity including asthma, coagulation defects, renal failure, severe heart failure or GI bleeding. Avoid in pregnancy.

Dose:

Ibuprofen, 300–400 mg q.d.s., p.o., to a max of 2.4 g daily.
Diclofenac, 25–50 mg t.d.s., p.o. or 75–150 mg o.d., p.r.

Opioids

Mechanism of action: Opioids act directly on the central nervous system, particularly in the pons and midbrain. There are three main types of opioid receptor:

- μ (mu receptors, found within the periaqueductal grey matter and are responsible for analgesia)
- δ (delta receptors, found within the periphery)
- κ (kappa receptors, found within the spinal cord).

1. Morphine

Morphine is predominantly a μ-receptor agonist. It is valuable for severe pain but has a broad range of side-effects. These range from nausea, vomiting, constipation, to eventually respiratory and cardiovascular depression at higher doses. It must be prescribed with care, especially in the elderly.

- Dose: 0.1–0.2 mg/kg.
- Start morphine as '**Immediate Release (IR) Morphine Sulphate (Oromorph)**' 4-hourly, p.o. In the young patient, 5–10 mg 4-hourly is often appropriate. In the elderly, or those with renal impairment, start at 2.5–5 mg 4-hourly.
- Associated with constipation, nausea and vomiting, and sedation. Co-prescribe the following, p.r.n.:
  — A **laxative**, e.g. lactulose 5–10 mL p.o. b.d.
  — An **antiemetic**, e.g. cyclizine 50 mg p.o. t.d.s.
  — An **opioid reversal agent** in case of sedation/overdose – **naloxone**, 100–400 micrograms i.v. every 5–10 minutes.
- Prescribe **1/6** of the total 24-hour opioid dose as required for **breakthrough** pain.

Review opioid dose frequently:

- If sedated/toxic – reduce dose.
- If pain controlled – continue same dose.
- If pain uncontrolled – calculate previous 24-hour total morphine

use, including p.r.n. doses. Recalculate 4-hourly requirement and prescribe at new dose. Do not increase by more than 50%. Adjust breakthrough dose accordingly.

Conversion to modified-release preparations

Modified release (MR) morphine allows less frequent dosing and a more even release of analgesia. When pain is controlled after 24 hours, you may convert to MR preparations by dividing the total 24 hours of Immediate Release dose by 2, and prescribing it as morphine sulphate MR b.d.

2. Opioid alternatives to morphine

a. *Codeine phosphate:* A weak opioid with a relatively low affinity for opioid receptors. The liver is responsible for demethylation of codeine to morphine.
   - Side-effects: nausea, constipation.
   - Dose: codeine phosphate, 30–60 mg q.d.s. p.o.

b. *Dihydrocodeine:* A semisynthetic opioid agonist related to codeine.
   - Side-effects: nausea, constipation.
   - Dose: Dihydrocodeine, 30 mg 4-hourly.

c. *Tramadol:* Mechanism of action is twofold. It is a weak μ-receptor agonist, and enhances serotonergic and adrenergic inhibitory pain pathways.
   - Side-effects: as with morphine.
   - Dose: Tramadol, 50–100 mg q.d.s., p.o./i.v./i.m.

d. *Pethidine:* Is a strong opioid that provides prompt but short-lived analgesia. Used during labour, in pancreatitis, and for perioperative pain.
   - Side-effects: as with morphine.
   - Dose: Pethidine, 50–150 mg, every 4 hours p.o.; *or* 25–100 mg, every 4 hours, i.m./s.c.

e. *Diamorphine:* Diacetylmorphine is the pro-drug of morphine. It has no clinical advantage over morphine but its high solubility makes it ideal for subcutaneous infusion and for combination with other drugs.

f. *Fentanyl:* Unlike morphine, fentanyl can be used in patients with renal failure. It can be delivered transdermally, as a patch (starting at 12 micrograms per hour) changed every 72 hours. This improves compliance and is effective for patients who cannot tolerate oral medication. The first patch will take 12–18 hours to provide maximal stable analgesia.

Contraindications and cautions: Caution in patients with impaired respiratory function, hypotension, obstructive or inflammatory bowel disorders, biliary tract disease, convulsive disorders and prostatic hypertrophy. Do not use in patients with acute respiratory depression, risk of paralytic ileus, raised intracranial pressure and head injury. Beware of tolerance and dependence.

Conversion of opioids

OPIOID	ROUTE	TYPICAL DOSE	24 HOUR MAX	RELATIVE TO ORAL MORPHINE DOSE
Codeine	p.o.	60 mg/4 hrs	240 mg	0.1
Dihydrocodeine	p.o.	30 mg/4 hrs	120 mg	0.1
Tramadol	p.o.	50 mg/4 hrs	600 mg	0.2
Morphine sulphate	p.o.	10 mg/1–4 hrs	N/A	1
Oxycodone	p.o.	5 mg/4 hrs	400 mg	2
Morphine	s.c./i.v./i.m.	5 mg/1–4 hrs	N/A	2
Diamorphine	s.c.	2.5 mg/1–4 hrs	N/A	3
Fentanyl patch	top.	25–75 micrograms/hr	2400 microgram	100–150

Adjuvant analgesics

Adjuvant analgesic drugs may be used alongside any step of the ladder. An adjuvant analgesic is a drug whose primary indication is for something other than pain, but which has analgesic effects in some painful conditions.

ADJUVANT ANALGESIC DRUGS	INDICATIONS
Corticosteroids	Nerve compression, raised intracranial pressure, liver capsular pain
Antidepressants and anticonvulsants	Neuropathic pain
Baclofen, benzodiazepines	Muscle cramps and spasms
Bisphosphonates	Bone pain

Adjuvant analgesia for neuropathic pain

These may be particularly effective for conditions such as chronic back pain, trigeminal neuralgia, and post-herpetic neuralgia. Non-pharmacological analgesia includes transcutaneous electrical nerve stimulation (TENS), acupuncture, cognitive behavioural therapy, and physiotherapy.

Tricyclic antidepressants

Examples: Amitriptyline.

Mechanism of action: At low doses, increases descending pain inhibitory pathway.

Side-effects: Antimuscarinic side-effects (including dry mouth, sedation, urinary retention) and cardiac side-effects (arrhythmias, hypotension).

Anticonvulsants

Examples: Carbamazepine, gabapentin.

Mechanism of action: Reduce depolarisation threshold.

Side-effects: Sedation, weight gain.

Patient-controlled analgesia (PCA)

PCA is an effective strategy for post-operative or severe continuous pain control if the patient is well enough to self-administer boluses when required. It allows for a continuous background infusion as maintenance.

Typical prescription:

- morphine 50 mg per 50 mL ready to use infusion
- bolus dose 1 mg i.v.

- lock-out 5 min
- background infusion 0 mg per hour
- **Naloxone, 100–400 micrograms, i.v., p.r.n. should always be co-prescribed.**

If the pain is not controlled, ask:

- Is it intermittent? If yes, increase bolus dose (max 3 mg).
- Is it constant? If yes, increase background infusion (max 3 mg/hr).
- **The bolus dose should be the same or more than the background rate.**

Palliative care

The dying patient may require end-of-life symptom control. Commonly, these symptoms include pain, dyspnoea, nausea and vomiting, respiratory tract secretions, and agitation/delirium.

The following drugs should be written up as p.r.n. unless there are specific contraindications. Anticipatory prescribing will ensure that in the last hours or days of life there is no delay in responding to symptoms if they occur.

MEDICATION	INDICATION	DOSE	ROUTE	FREQUENCY
Morphine	Pain Dyspnoea	2.5–5 mg	s.c.	p.r.n. (max 1-hrly)
Metoclopramide	Nausea and Vomiting	10 mg	s.c.	p.r.n. (max 6-hrly)
Haloperidol	Agitation/Delirium	1.5–5 mg	s.c.	p.r.n. (max 8-hrly)
Midazolam	Restlessness/ Agitation Terminal Dyspnoea	2.5–5 mg	s.c.	p.r.n. (max 1-hrly)
Glycopyrronium bromide	Secretions	200 micrograms	s.c.	p.r.n. (max 4-hrly)

Patients with symptoms refractory to regular p.r.n. doses may require medication given by continuous subcutaneous infusion, via a syringe driver. Never mix more than three drugs in a syringe driver unless advised by a palliative care team. Remember to place a second subcutaneous butterfly to avoid repeated injections for additional p.r.n. doses.

Indications for starting a continuous subcutaneous infusion include the following.

- *Pain* – if a patient requires more than 3 p.r.n. doses each day.
- *Dyspnoea* – if a patient has a strong anxiety component responsive to midazolam p.r.n.
- *Nausea and vomiting* – if a patient has constant nausea and vomiting or requires more than 2 doses of p.r.n. antiemetic.
- *Respiratory tract secretions* – if a patient has continuous secretions uncontrolled by glycopyrronium.
- *Restlessness and agitation* – if a patient requires more than 3 p.r.n. doses of midazolam each day.

Consult local guidelines for exact dosing for syringe drivers.

Reference

National Health Service. *Palliative Care Guidelines*. NECN Palliative Care Clinical Group: North of England Cancer Network; 2010.

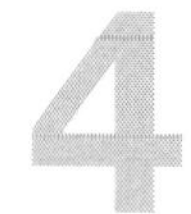

Antiemetics

Antiemetics are commonly used to target nausea and vomiting. The choice of antiemetic can be dependent upon the cause of nausea. If adequately prescribed, they can significantly reduce morbidity.

Physiology

The perception of nausea and vomiting can be due to the activation of receptors throughout the body:

- gut and central nervous system (CNS) chemo- and pressure-receptors
- peripheral pain receptors
- the chemoreceptor trigger zone (CTZ), which is located near the fourth ventricle. Raised intracranial pressure is thought to contribute to nausea and vomiting through a pressure effect in this area. This area is also susceptible to emetogenic chemotherapy agents and morphine.

The vomiting centre is located in the reticular formation of the medulla and is responsible for the initiation and control of the vomiting reflex via brainstem nuclei.

A number of neurotransmitters are responsible for nausea and vomiting. Pharmacological control of nausea and vomiting is based upon antagonising these mechanisms.

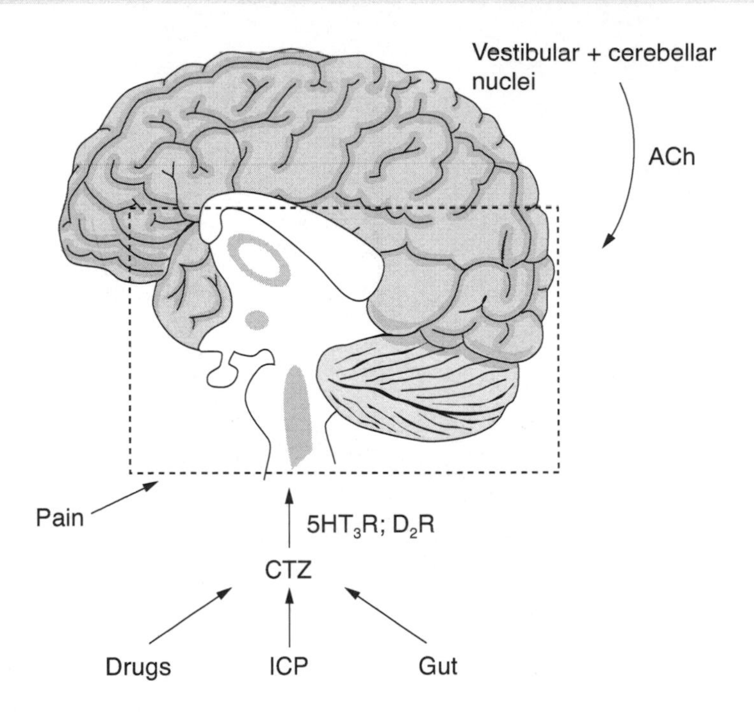

A. Histamine antagonists

Mechanism of action: Work primarily upon vestibular nuclei, which mediate their action via histamine and acetylcholine receptors.

Indications:

- motion sickness (and labyrinthitis)
- post-operative nausea and vomiting
- opioid analgesic-related nausea and vomiting.

Examples: Cyclizine (competitive H_1 antagonist).

Dose: Cyclizine, 50 mg, p.o./i.v./i.m., t.d.s.

B. $5HT_3$ (serotonergic) antagonists

Mechanism of action: Highly-selective $5HT_3$ antagonists. These receptors are found in high quantities in the CTZ.

Indications:

- post-operative nausea and vomiting (PONV)
- cytotoxic/chemotherapy-induced vomiting.

Example: Ondansetron.

Dose: Ondansetron 4–8 mg p.o./i.v./i.m., t.d.s.

C. Dopamine receptor (D_2R) antagonists

Mechanism of action: Dopamine receptor antagonist at the CTZ. It is indicated for nausea and vomiting of gastric stasis, e.g. due to ascites, hepatomegaly, mesenteric nodes, opioids or functional/partial obstruction.

Indications:

- gastrointestinal emesis.

Examples: Metoclopramide, domperidone.

Contraindications and cautions: Due to the blockade of other dopamine receptors in the CNS, metoclopramide can lead to CNS side-effects. In children and young adults, the patient can become fatigued, or in severe cases can experience extrapyramidal effects (oculogyric crises or spasmodic torticollis). Domperidone does not cross the blood–brain barrier and hence is less likely to cause central effects. These are contraindicated in gastrointestinal obstruction.

Dose:
Metoclopramide 10 mg p.o./i.v./i.m., t.d.s.
Domperidone 10 mg p.o., q.d.s.

D. Phenothiazines

Mechanism of action: These are dopamine D_2 antagonists at the CTZ.

Indications:

- terminal illness
- schizophrenia
- hiccups
- labyrinthine illness.

Examples: Prochlorperazine, chlorpromazine.

Contraindications and cautions: Like metoclopramide, chlorpromazine use can lead to extrapyramidal side-effects. Prochlorperazine is less sedating than chlorpromazine, and can be given by i.m. injection or rectal suppository if the patient is vomiting.

Dose: Prochlorperazine 5–10 mg p.o. t.d.s.

E. Anti-cholinergics

Mechanism of action: Acetylcholine (ACh) receptor antagonists.

Indications:

- motion sickness/vomiting arising from vestibular nuclei (takes 1–2 hours to peak after ingestion); most useful when taken prophylactically
- premedication for anaesthesia.

Examples: Hyoscine hydrobromide.

Dose: Hyoscine hydrobromide 150–300 micrograms p.o., q.d.s.

F. Dexamethasone

The antiemetic mechanism of action is unclear. It is useful for nausea and vomiting of metastatic disease and for PONV.

Dose: Dexamethasone 8 mg i.v., o.d.

Reference

Anaesthesia UK. *Nausea and Vomiting*. 2004. Available online at: www.frca.co.uk/SectionContents.aspx?sectionid=113 (accessed 8 May 2012).

5

Fluids

Total body water is approximately 60% total body weight. A 70 kg man is therefore composed of 42 L water.

Total body fluid = 60% of body mass 42 L

Two-thirds of the total body water is intracellular, and one-third is extracellular.

Intracellular volume = 40% of body mass 28 L	Extracellular volume = 20% of body mass 14 L

The extracellular fluid is split into interstitial fluid (10 L), plasma (3 L) and transcellular fluid (1 L).

Interstitial fluid (10 L)	Plasma (3 L)	Transcellular fluid (1 L)

Adequate fluid management involves water and electrolyte replacement. Daily electrolyte requirements are as follows:

- Na^+: 70–150 mmol
- K^+: 40–70 mmol

Types of fluid

1. Crystalloids

a. 'Normal' 0.9% saline

This is an isotonic crystalloid containing 154 mmol/L Na^{+}. When infused, it diffuses throughout the extracellular fluid compartment. After 30 minutes, 25% of the fluid remains intravascular. Despite this it may be used as a resuscitation fluid. Prolonged use can lead to hyperchloraemic metabolic acidosis and sodium overload, and caution must be taken in patients with cirrhotic liver disease.

b. Five per cent dextrose

This is a hypotonic crystalloid. Once the glucose is metabolised by the liver, free water remains. This is rapidly distributed throughout the extracellular fluid compartment *and* intracellular fluid compartment. Consequently, after 30 minutes, only approximately 10% remains intravascular. This makes 5% dextrose a poor fluid for use in resuscitation; however, it is good for sustaining hydration. Overuse can lead to hyponatraemia.

c. Hartmann's solution

This is a crystalloid, and is thought to be the most 'physiological'. It is the most common perioperative fluid used. It contains lactate and so should be avoided in diabetic ketoacidosis and used with caution in cirrhotic liver disease.

2. Colloid

Intravascular volume is determined by:

- permeability of blood vessels
- hydrostatic pressure
- oncotic pressure.

Oncotic pressure is the ability of a fluid to retain water in circulation, and is brought about by the presence of albumin, haemoglobin and globulins (of which albumin contributes around 70%). Colloids are fluids that increase the oncotic pressure of intravascular fluid, which helps to expand intravascular volume. These fluids are beneficial in major haemorrhage and severe sepsis. Side-effects include itching, bleeding and anaphylaxis.

Fluid composition

		Na^+ (mmol/L)	K^+ (mmol/L)	Ca^{2+} (mmol/L)	Cl^- (mmol/L)	HCO^-_3 (mmol/L)	pH	Osmolality (mosmol/L)
Crystalloid	0.9% NaCl	154	0	0	154	0	5.5	300
	Hartmann's	131	5	4	112	29	6.5	281
	5% glucose	0	0	0	0	0	4.1	278
Colloid	Gelofusine	154	0.4	0.4	125	0	7.4	465

Maintenance fluids

A normal adult loses approximately 2.5–3 L of water per day, together with 70–150 mmol of Na^+ and 60 mmol of K^+.

Maintenance fluids replace ongoing losses. An apyrexial patient with no excess losses (e.g. via drains or gastrointestinal losses) can be estimated as follows:

- **For the first 10 kg: 4 mL/kg/hr.**
- **For the next 10 kg: 2 mL/kg/hr.**
- **For every kg above 20 kg: 1 mL/kg/hr.**

For a 70 kg adult this equates to 2.5 L/day. Over 30 hours, it can be prescribed as follows:

- **1 L 0.9% saline + 20 mmol/L K^+ i.v. over 10 hours.**
- **1 L 5% dextrose + 20 mmol/L K^+ i.v. over 10 hours.**
- **1 L 5% dextrose + 20 mmol/L K^+ i.v. over 10 hours.**

Conditions with specific fluid requirements

Certain conditions have specific fluid requirements, as discussed below.

Hypovolaemic shock

Shock can be classified into four types by signs and symptoms. Crystalloid is appropriate fluid resuscitation for Class I and II but Class III and IV require crystalloid and/or blood.

	CLASS I	CLASS II	CLASS III	CLASS IV
Blood loss (mL)	≤750	750–1500	1500–2000	≥2000
Blood loss (% blood volume)	≤15	15–30	30–40	≥40
Pulse rate (per min)	<100	>100	>120	≥140
Blood pressure	Normal	Normal	Decreased	Decreased
Pulse pressure	Normal or increased	Decreased	Decreased	Decreased
Capillary refill test	Normal	Positive	Positive	Positive
Respiratory rate (breaths × min^{-1})	14–20	20–30	30–40	<35
Urine output (mL × hr^{-1})	≥30	20–30	5–15	Negligible
CNS mental status	Slightly anxious	Mildly anxious	Anxious and confused	Confused, lethargic
Fluid replacement (3:1 rule)	Crystalloid	Crystalloid	Crystalloid + blood	Crystalloid + blood

Gastrointestinal losses

It is important to quantify the amount of fluid loss by taking a detailed history. The fluid deficit must be replaced, followed by continued maintenance fluid if the patient continues to vomit despite medical intervention. Prolonged vomiting can lead to hypochloraemic hypokalaemic metabolic alkalosis, requiring appropriate potassium replacement.

Post-operative patients

Many patients can be dehydrated post-operatively despite adequate fluid resuscitation. This can be due to:

- prolonged pre-operative fasting
- intraoperative losses (e.g. via heat, lungs or blood)
- fluid shift into the physiological third-space.

If post-operative blood pressure remains low despite adequate fluid resuscitation, Hartmann's solution can be infused (at twice the maintenance infusion rate). If this fails, colloid fluid challenges may be required to maintain the circulation.

Colloid fluid challenge

This is a rapid administration of intravenous fluid given in a state of hypoperfusion. It is often used to detect hypovolaemia. A 10% or more rise in cardiac output indicates relative hypovolaemia. The volume of a fluid challenge should be appropriately reduced in patients with heart failure.

e.g. 500 mL Gelofusine i.v. stat

Remember, if hypotension remains a problem despite these measures, the patient may be bleeding internally and requires urgent escalation.

Sepsis

Sepsis is defined as 'systemic inflammatory response syndrome' (SIRS) with evidence of infection. The SIRS criteria are as follows:

Any two out of:

- tachycardia (>90 beats per minute)
- respiratory rate (>20 breaths per minute) or $PaCO_2$ <4.3 kPa
- temperature (<36°C or >38°C)
- white cell count (<4 or >10 × 10^9/L).

During sepsis, increased vascular permeability leads to leakage of plasma proteins and fluid, reducing the circulating volume. Initially, Hartmann's solution or colloid can be given to raise the blood pressure, and continuous monitoring is required to ensure that the patient's conscious level does not deteriorate and that the patient is maintaining adequate urine output (>0.5 mL/kg/hr). This may require a urinary catheter.

If the patient does not respond to these measures, and is a candidate for intensive care, they would require invasive blood pressure monitoring (such as central venous pressure and arterial lines).

Fluid balance charts

The use of a fluid balance chart in coordination with daily weights on the ward, a daily clinical assessment of fluid status and the laboratory assessment of urea, electrolytes and fluid balance help the clinician understand whether the patient is over- or under-hydrated. These charts must be completed carefully and in detail, as some patients require careful fluid administration.

The cumulative balance is important to calculate. In a patient that is dehydrated (and is already in a state analogous to a negative fluid balance), the aim would be to create a 'positive balance'. Conversely, in a patient that is fluid overloaded (e.g. due to liver or cardiac failure), one would aim to create a 'negative balance'.

TIME	**INPUT (mL)**				**OUTPUT (mL)**							
	Oral	i.v.	Nutrition	**Total**	Urine	Naso-Gastric	Vomit	Bowel/ Stoma	Drains	**Total**	2 hourly Balance +/–	**Cumulative Balance +/–**
0600	–	–	–	–	400	–	–	–	–	400	–400	**–400**
0800	–	500	–	500	100	–	–	–	–	100	+400	**0**
1000	50	500	–	550	50	–	50	–	–	100	+450	**+450**
1200	–	100	100	200	375	–	150	–	–	225	–25	**+425**
1400	–	50	–	50	250	–	50	–	–	200	–150	**+275**
1600	50	–	–	50	75	–	–	–	–	75	–25	**+250**
1800	75	–	150	225	50	–	–	–	–	50	+175	**+425**
2000	–	–	–	–	50	–	–	–	–	50	–50	**+375**

References

Leach R. Fluid management on hospital medical wards. *Clin Med.* 2010 Dec; **10**(6): 611–15.

Mackenzie I. Fluid and electrolyte balance, anaemia and blood transfusion. *Surgery.* 2005; **23**(12): 453–60.

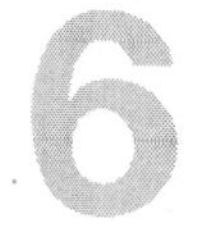

Thromboprophylaxis and anticoagulation

The coagulation cascade

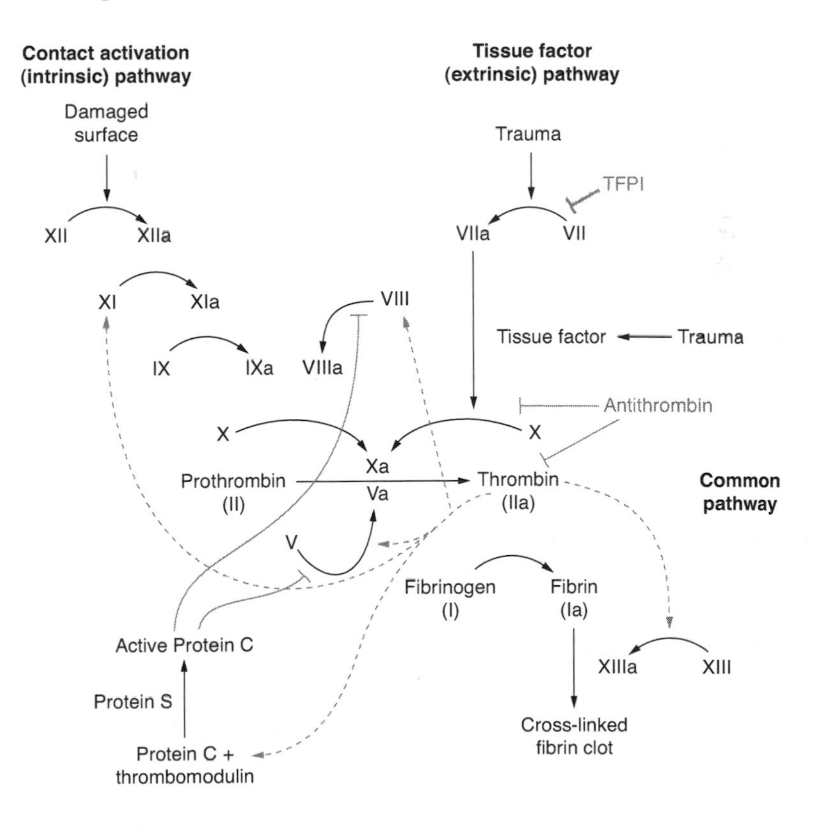

Two pathways lead to fibrin formation: the intrinsic and extrinsic pathways. Physiologically, both pathways lead to the formation of thrombin from prothrombin, which requires factor Xa. Thrombin is responsible for the conversion of fibrinogen to fibrin, which in turn leads to a cross-linked fibrin clot.

- **Prothrombin time (PT):** This is a measure of the extrinsic pathway, which can be prolonged in vitamin K deficiency, warfarin use or malabsorption.
- **International normalised ratio (INR):** Due to laboratory variation in calculating PT, the concept of INR has been developed to standardise prothrombin time. This is calculated as a ratio of the patient's PT to PT of a control sample. A normal INR ranges from 0.8 to 1.2.
- **Activated partial thromboplastin time (APTT):** This is a measure of the intrinsic pathway, and is used to measure the effect of unfractionated heparin.

Venous thromboembolism and heparin

Venous thromboembolism (VTE) is a term encompassing deep vein thrombosis (DVT) and pulmonary embolus (PE). Up to one in five patients undergoing major surgery (and up to two in five undergoing orthopaedic surgery) can experience DVT. Consequently, there is a need for thromboprophylaxis in hospitalised patients.

VTE prophylaxis can be mechanical prophylaxis (such as compression stockings) or pharmacological prophylaxis (heparins). In addition, patients should be well hydrated and mobilise as soon as possible.

Low molecular weight heparin

Low molecular weight heparin (LMWH), including dalteparin and enoxaparin, has the advantage over unfractionated heparins as it does not require daily monitoring of APTT. LMWH potentiates the anti-Xa activity of antithrombin. The dose of LMWH should be reduced appropriately in patients with chronic renal failure.

On admission to hospital, every patient must have a thrombotic risk assessment:

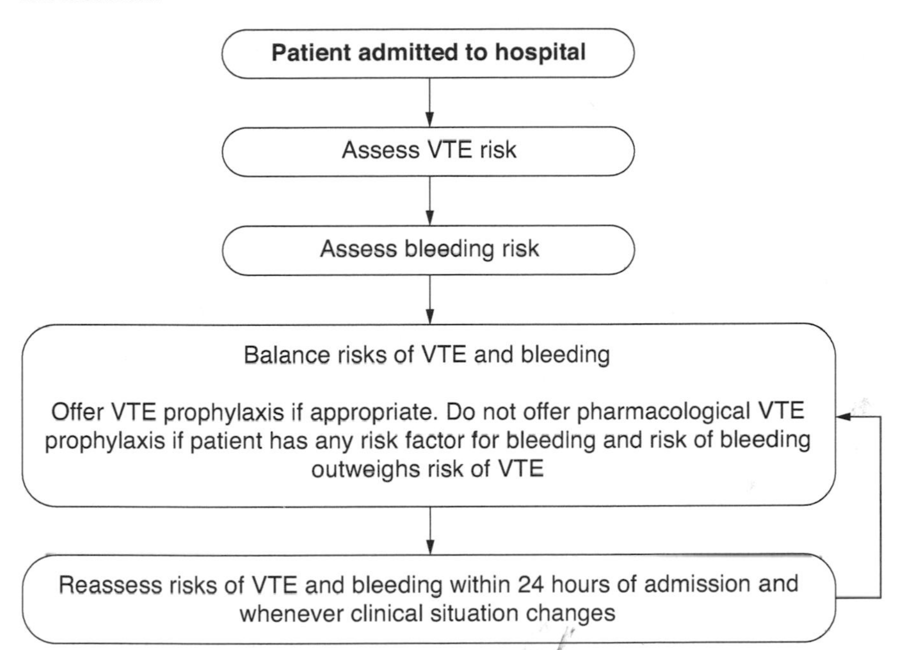

Patients at risk of VTE

PATIENTS WHO ARE AT RISK OF VTE	
Medical patients If mobility significantly reduced for ≥3 days **or** If expected to have ongoing reduced mobility relative to normal state plus any VTE risk factor	**Surgical patients and patients with trauma** • If total anaesthetic + surgical time >90 minutes **or** • If surgery involves pelvis or lower limb and total anaesthetic + surgical time >60 minutes **or** • If acute surgical admission with inflammatory or intra-abdominal condition **or** • If expected to have significant reduction in mobility **or** • If any VTE risk factor present

(*continued*)

PATIENTS WHO ARE AT RISK OF VTE

VTE risk factors

- Active cancer or cancer treatment
- Age >60 years
- Critical care admission
- Dehydration
- Known thrombophilias
- Obesity (BMI >30 kg/m^2)
- One or more significant medical comorbidities (e.g. heart disease; metabolic, endocrine or respiratory pathologies; acute infectious diseases; inflammatory conditions)
- Personal history or first-degree relative with a history of VTE
- Use of HRT
- Use of oestrogen-containing contraceptive therapy
- Varicose veins with phlebitis

After assessment of risk, contraindications to thromboprophylaxis must be assessed, as follows.

PATIENTS WHO ARE AT RISK OF BLEEDING

All patients who have any of the following:

- Active bleeding
- Acquired bleeding disorders (e.g. acute liver failure)
- Concurrent use of anticoagulants known to increase the risk of bleeding (e.g. warfarin with INR >2)
- Lumbar puncture/epidural/spinal anaesthesia within the previous 4 hours or expected within the next 12 hours
- Acute stroke
- Thrombocytopaenia (platelets $<75 \times 10^9$/L)
- Uncontrolled systolic hypertension (≥230/120 mmHg)
- Untreated inherited bleeding disorders (such as haemophilia or von Willebrand disease)

Anti-embolism stockings

Do not offer anti-embolism stockings to patients with:

- suspected or proven peripheral arterial disease
- peripheral arterial bypass grafting
- peripheral neuropathy or other causes of sensory impairment

- local condition in which stockings may cause damage, such as fragile skin, dermatitis, gangrene or recent skin graft
- known allergy to material
- cardiac failure
- severe leg oedema or pulmonary oedema from congestive heart failure
- unusual leg size or shape
- major limb deformity preventing correct fit.

Use caution and clinical judgement when applying anti-embolism stockings over venous ulcers or wounds.

Example prescription

DALTEPARIN | 5000 units | s.c. | o.d. |

Direct thrombin inhibitors, such as lepirudin and argatroban may be used instead of heparins in a small proportion of patients who experience heparin-induced thrombocytopaenia.

Treatment of DVT/PE

Deep vein thrombosis (DVT) occurs most commonly in the leg veins. It is characterised by unilateral leg pain, oedema and swelling.

Pulmonary embolus (PE) is characterised by tachypnoea, tachycardia, haemoptysis, hypotension and focal chest signs. For a PE, computed tomography pulmonary angiogram is the first line radiological investigation, unless contraindicated.

A massive PE is treated by thrombolysis (e.g. alteplase – a tissue plasminogen activator); however, a non-massive PE can be treated with heparins and prevented with anticoagulation.

Commencing anticoagulation using **warfarin** will require concurrent initial *treatment* dose of **low molecular weight heparin**. LMWH should be continued for **5 days or until the INR has been greater than or equal to 2.0 for 24 hours – whichever is longer**.

Concurrent use of warfarin and LMWH is required because of the following.

1. Warfarin has an initial prothrombotic effect.
2. Warfarin is a vitamin K antagonist. It therefore depletes vitamin-K dependent clotting factors, including Factor II (prothrombin). Factor II has a half-life of 50 hours in patients with normal hepatic clearance. Warfarin does not reach full therapeutic effect until after 5 days.

The target **INR is 2–3**, and treatment is for 6 weeks for a below knee DVT or 3–6 months for an above knee DVT or PE.

Treatment dose of dalteparin

Under 46 kg	7500 units daily
46–56 kg	10 000 units daily
57–68 kg	12 500 units daily
69–82 kg	15 000 units daily
83–120 kg	18 000 units daily
000 units	

+ concurrent warfarin.

Warfarin

Warfarin is a vitamin K antagonist. It acts by inhibiting the reductase enzyme responsible for synthesising the active form of vitamin K. It therefore reduces the levels of vitamin K-dependent clotting factors, namely II, VII, IX and X.

Vitamin K antagonists comprise of:

- coumarins (such as warfarin and acenocoumarol)
- indanediones (such as phenindione).

The main **indications for vitamin K antagonists** are:

- prevention of venous thromboembolism

- prevention of systemic embolism (e.g. stroke)
- in patients with mechanical heart valves
- in patients with atrial fibrillation
- prophylaxis against systemic embolism following myocardial infarction.

The **absolute contraindications for anticoagulation** are:

- potential bleeding lesions
- active peptic ulcer, oesophageal varices, aneurysm and proliferative retinopathy
- recent organ biopsy
- recent trauma or surgery to the head, orbit or spine
- recent stroke
- confirmed intracranial or intraspinal bleed
- uncontrolled hypertension
- infective endocarditis.

The various indications have different target INRs to minimise the risk of thromboembolism as follows.

INDICATION	TARGET INR	DURATION OF ANTICOAGULATION
Pulmonary embolus	2.5	Six months
Proximal deep vein thrombosis	2.5	Six months
Calf vein thrombosis	2.5	Three months
Recurrence of venous thromboembolism when no longer on warfarin	2.5	Consider long term
Recurrence of venous thromboembolism while on warfarin	3.5	Consider long term
Antiphospholipid syndrome	2.5	Consider long term
Atrial fibrillation	2.5	Long term

(*continued*)

INDICATION	TARGET INR	DURATION OF ANTICOAGULATION
Cardioversion	2.5 or 3.0	Three weeks before and four weeks after procedure
Mural thrombus	2.5	Three months
Cardiomyopathy	2.5	Long term
Mechanical prosthetic heart valve*	2.5 or 3.0	Long term

* *Aortic* mechanical prosthetic heart valves have a target INR of 2.5–3.0. *Mitral* mechanical prosthetic heart valves have a target INR of 3.0–3.5.

Initiating oral anticoagulation

Test for the patient's baseline INR. If it is greater than 1.4, screen for coagulopathies.

LMWH is predominantly excreted by the kidneys. In patients with renal failure (creatinine clearance <30 mL/min) there is a danger of accumulation. In this situation, **unfractionated heparin** is the treatment of choice.

LMWH should be continued for **5 days or until the INR has been greater than or equal to 2.0 for 24 hours - whichever is longer**.

> Blood bottles for clotting come pre-filled with citrate. High citrate levels will give spuriously high INRs. Fill the sample bottles to the top and do not pour two small samples into one bottle to make up volume!

The regimen for initiating warfarin may vary between hospitals.

For example: A starting dose of **5 mg warfarin p.o.** is to be given for the first two days. The INR is checked on the mornings of **days 3 and 4**, and the warfarin dose is adjusted accordingly. An example regimen table, aiming for INR 2–3, is shown here:

DAYS 1 & 2	DAY 3		DAY 4	
	INR	Dose	INR	Dose
Give 5 mg each evening if baseline INR less than or equal to 1.3	<1.5	10 mg	<1.6	10 mg
	1.5–2.0	5 mg	1.6–1.7	7 mg
	2.1–2.5	3 mg	1.8–1.9	6 mg
	2.6–3.0	1 mg	2.0–2.3	5 mg
	>3.0	0 mg	2.4–2.7	4 mg
			2.8–3.0	3 mg
			3.1–3.5	2 mg
			3.6–4.0	1 mg
			>4.0	0 mg

The dose **at day 4** is a good predictor of the maintenance dose in most patients. All patients should be referred to an anticoagulant clinic as soon as possible after commencement of warfarin, where they can be advised further regarding monitoring INR and dosing their warfarin. At discharge, ensure that the following are performed.

1. Confirm anticoagulant clinic follow-up, which should be within 48 hours of discharge.
2. The discharge documentation should include:
   a. indication for starting oral anticoagulation
   b. target INR
   c. duration of therapy.

Note that warfarin interacts with many medications, supplements and foods.

Reversal of oral anticoagulation

Vitamin K (phytomenadione)

Vitamin K is absorbed from the small intestine and stored in the liver. It controls haemostasis by regulating the vitamin K-dependent clotting factors II, VII, IX and X. These clotting factors promote the formation of fibrin, via the clotting cascade. In anticoagulated patients, only a small amount of vitamin K is required to promote the production of clotting factors and reverse anticoagulation.

Prothrombin complex concentrate (PCC)

PCCs, such as Beriplex and Octaplex, contain three or four vitamin K-dependent clotting factors. They may also contact vitamin K-dependent coagulation inhibitors Protein C and Protein S. PCCs normalise the levels of vitamin K-dependent clotting factors to re-establish haemostasis.

Patients may need reversal of their anticoagulation temporarily (e.g. active bleeding, prior to undergoing surgery, or interactions with new medications) or permanently (e.g. liver failure).

The risk of bleeding while on warfarin increases significantly with INR levels above 4.5. Patients who are over-anticoagulated may therefore also need reversal.

A. Major bleeding (regardless of INR)

Patients with intracranial or rapid-onset neurological signs, intra-ocular bleeds, compartment syndrome, pericardial bleeds or those with active bleeding and shock need urgent assessment of clotting.

1. Check INR and APTT and FBC.
2. Stop warfarin.
3. Reverse anticoagulation with 30 units/kg prothrombin complex concentrate i.v. up to maximum dose 3000 units.
4. Reverse anticoagulation with 5–10 mg vitamin K i.v.
5. Recheck coagulation screen and full blood count.

B. Minor bleeding with INR 5.0 or more

1. Check INR and APTT and FBC.
2. **Omit** warfarin.
3. Give 5–10 mg vitamin K i.v.

C. Minor bleeding with INR <5.0

1. Check INR and APTT and FBC.
2. Make a clinical decision whether lowering the INR is required.

3. Consider giving 0.5–1.0 mg vitamin K i.v. and modifying warfarin dose.

D. No bleeding with INR 5.0–7.9

1. **Omit** warfarin.
2. Restart at a lower dose when INR <5.0.

E. No bleeding with INR 8.0–12.0

1. **Omit** warfarin.
2. Give 2 mg oral vitamin K.

F. No bleeding with INR >12.0

1. **Omit** warfarin.
2. Give 5 mg oral vitamin K.

References

British Thoracic Society guidelines for the management of suspected acute pulmonary embolism. *Thorax* 2003; **58**(6): 470–3.

National Institute for Health and Clinical Excellence. *Venous Thromboembolism: reducing the risk*: NICE Guideline 92. London: NIHCE; 2010. www.nice.org.uk/guidance/CG92

7

Constipation

Symptoms

- Hard faeces, which are uncomfortable or difficult to pass; reduced frequency compared with normal pattern.
- Sense of incomplete evacuation after defecation.
- Colicky abdominal pain, flatulence, distension.
- Nausea, vomiting, anorexia, malaise, headache and halitosis.
- Constipation may lead to urinary retention and frequency.
- Overflow diarrhoea.

Causes

- ***Disease related:*** Immobility, reduced food intake/low residue diet, intra-abdominal and pelvic disease.
- ***Fluid depletion:*** Poor fluid intake/increased fluid loss, e.g. vomiting, fever, fistula output and excessively exudative wounds.
- ***Weakness:*** Inability to raise intra-abdominal pressure, e.g. paraplegia/general debility.
- ***Intestinal obstruction:*** Disease presentation or recurrence, adhesions.

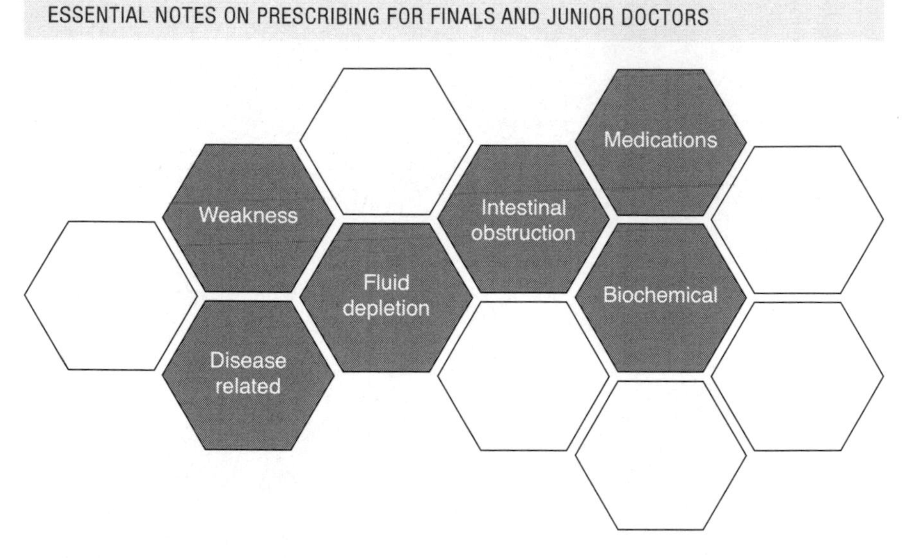

- ***Medications:*** Especially opioids, diuretics, phenothiazines, anticholinergic drugs (e.g. tricyclic antidepressants and hyoscine salts), $5HT_3$ antagonists.
- ***Biochemical:*** Hypercalcaemia, hypokalaemia.
- ***Other:*** Embarrassment, pain on defecation.

Management

- Attempt to increase fluid/fibre intake and encourage mobility.
- Use a combination of laxatives with different mechanisms of action as appropriate.
- Titrate laxative to achieve optimal stool frequency and consistency.

Commonly used laxatives

CATEGORY	EXAMPLES	DESCRIPTION	EXAMPLE DOSAGE
Osmotic laxatives	Lactulose Movicol	Not absorbed from the gut. Retain water in the lumen thus increasing volume, peristalsis and expulsion of faeces	**Lactulose** 15 mL b.d. p.o. **Movicol** Start with 1–3 sachets/day
Stool softeners	Liquid paraffin Arachis oil Docusate	Reduce surface tension and improve water penetration of stools	**Liquid paraffin** 10–30 mL at night **Arachis oil** 130 mL (warmed) enema **Docusate** 100–200 mg b.d./t.d.s.
Bulk-forming laxatives	Ispaghula husk Bran	Increase faecal mass to stimulate peristalsis	**Fybogel** 1 sachet b.d.
Stimulant laxatives	Senna Bisacodyl Sodium picosulphate	Increase intestinal motility and often cause abdominal cramp. Excess use can cause diarrhoea and hypokalaemia	**Senna** 1–2 tablets BD
Combined stimulant & softening laxatives	Co-danthramer		1–2 capsules at bedtime
Suppositories	Glycerin Bisacodyl Phosphate enema	Glycerin and bisacodyl are stimulant p.r. laxatives. Phosphate enemas are p.r. osmotic laxatives	

Uses

Acute use in the non-obstructed patient

- Senna 1–2 tablets p.o. b.d. *or*
- Glycerin or bisacodyl p.r. suppositories.
- Consider docusate 100 mg t.d.s. if necessary.

Impaction and overflow

- Phosphate enema 1 p.r. suppository.
- Follow if necessary with arachis oil enema or glycerine p.r. suppository.
- Movicol can be used where the above has failed.
- Sodium citrate micro-enema can be used but is usually reserved for pre-procedural bowel preparation.
- Consider manual evacuation if enema fails.

Chronic constipation (prevention)

- Ispaghula husk (e.g. Fybogel) 1 sachet b.d. p.o. *or*
- Docusate 100 mg capsules t.d.s. p.o.

Terminally ill patients

- Co-danthramer 1–3 capsules p.o. nocte.

Opiate-induced constipation

- Senna 1–2 tablets p.o. nocte.
- Consider docusate 100 mg capsules p.o., t.d.s. if necessary.

Bowel preparation

Bowel-cleansing agents, including Picolax, Klean-Prep and Citrafleet, should not be used to treat constipation.

These agents are commonly used to prepare the bowel prior to colonic surgery or colonoscopy to ensure the bowel can be examined fully. However, they should be used with caution in patients with renal dysfunction, electrolyte imbalance, hypovolaemia and colitis. They are contraindicated in patients with gastrointestinal obstruction or perforation, acute severe colitis or toxic megacolon.

A common bowel-preparation regime is shown on page 59. However, consult hospital guidelines prior to prescribing bowel-preparation on the wards.

No food after breakfast the day before procedure
Clear fluids only

Magnesium citrate
1 sachet at 4 p.m. on evening before procedure
1 sachet at 8 p.m. on evening before procedure

Antidiarrhoeals

Codeine phosphate and loperamide are antidiarrhoeals with an opioid action. They act at mu-receptors in myenteric plexus to reduce acetylcholine release, and therefore peristalsis. They also increase anal tone. Loperamide does not cross the blood–brain barrier, and is therefore preferred.

Codeine phosphate, 15–60 mg, p.o., max q.d.s.

or

Loperamide hydrochloride, 2–4 mg, p.o., max 16 mg/day

8

Diabetes mellitus

Type 1 diabetes mellitus presents mostly in young patients, and is usually caused by autoimmune destruction of insulin-producing beta cells in the pancreas.

Type 2 diabetes mellitus is usually a disorder of background insulin insensitivity with a failure of compensatory pancreatic insulin secretion, and is seen in older patients. While Type 2 diabetes mellitus is not insulin-dependent, many people eventually require insulin for optimal blood glucose control.

Diabetes mellitus is notable for associated increased cardiovascular risk, manifested as coronary artery disease, peripheral artery disease and carotid artery disease.

Patients may present with:

- polyuria
- thirst
- weight loss
- fatigue.

Poor control can result in hyperosmolar coma (particularly in Type 2 diabetes mellitus) and diabetic ketoacidosis (more common in Type 1 diabetes mellitus).

Blood glucose and HbA_{1c}

Raised fasting blood glucose of greater than 11.1 mmol/L is indicative of diabetes and is confirmed by the oral glucose tolerance test. Glycosuria can raise the suspicion of diabetes but is not diagnostic.

HbA_{1c} concentration allows monitoring of diabetes. Haemoglobin A (HbA) reacts non-enzymatically with glucose in the bloodstream in a concentration-dependent manner. HbA remains in the circulation for approximately 3 months. HbA_{1c} is the predominant form of glycated haemoglobin, and, when expressed as a percentage of HbA is proportional to blood glucose concentrations over the previous 3 months. Current guidelines suggest aiming for HbA_{1c} <6.5%.

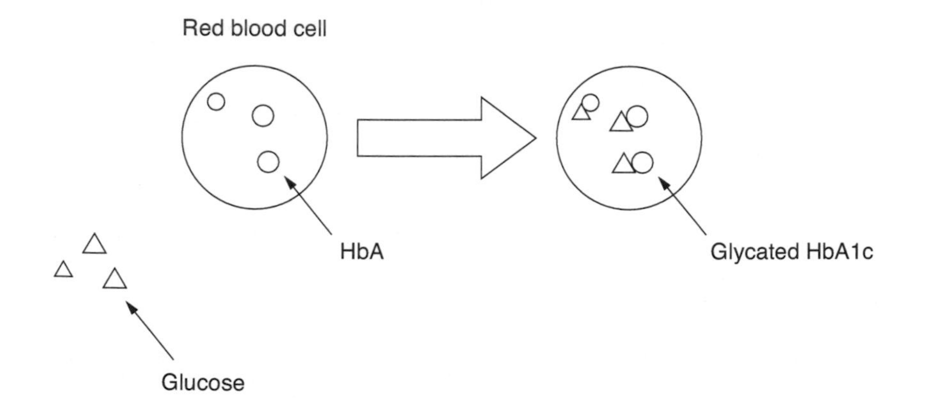

Treatment of diabetes mellitus

General measures:

- education and lifestyle changes
- maintain blood pressure <140/80 mmHg or <130/80 mmHg in those with diabetic microvascular complications; ACE-inhibitors are first line antihypertensives.

Non-insulin anti-diabetic medication

A. Biguanides

Mechanism of action: Improve sensitivity to insulin. There is no risk of hypoglycaemia. Biguanides also lower fasting insulin levels by inducing greater peripheral uptake of glucose, and decrease hepatic glucose output.

Example: Metformin.
Used as first line for overweight patients where blood glucose levels are not controlled by lifestyle changes alone.

Contraindications:

- **Renal disease:** Metformin is excreted unchanged in the urine. Accumulation can result in life-threatening lactic acidosis. Patients with renal disease, evidenced by elevated serum creatinine (>130 micromol/L) or reduced eGFR (<45 mL/min/1.73 m^2) should have their dose carefully reviewed. Patients with sepsis, dehydration or shock can have impaired renal function and should have their metformin reviewed.
- Iodinated contrasts: Metformin should be withheld for 24–48 hours before patients undergo imaging investigations using iodinated contrast agents, such as CT angiograms. Metformin should be recommenced 48 hours afterwards and only when renal function is shown to be normal.

Common and important side-effects: Life-threatening lactic acidosis, nausea and vomiting.

B. Secretagogues

i. Sulphonylureas

Mechanism of action: Stimulate pancreatic insulin release. These are used as first line if:

- patient is not overweight, *or*
- cannot tolerate metformin, *or*
- requires a rapid response to therapy due to hyperglycaemic symptoms.

Sulphonylurea is added as second line if glucose control is not adequate with metformin.

Examples: Gliclazide, glimepiride, tolbutamide.

Common and important side-effects: Weight gain, hypoglycaemia.

ii. Rapid-acting insulin secretagogues

Mechanism of action: Stimulate pancreatic insulin release. These are considered for a person with an erratic lifestyle.

Examples: Nateglinide, repaglinide.

iii. Alpha-glucosidase inhibitors

Mechanism of action: Reduces the rate of digestion of complex carbohydrates by the enzyme alpha-glucosidase. These are considered in patients who cannot use any other oral glucose-lowering medication.

Examples: Acarbose.

Common and important side-effects: Flatulence, diarrhoea. Hepatitis has been reported, and therefore liver function tests must be monitored regularly in patients taking acarbose.

iv. Thiazolidinedione (glitazones)

Mechanism of action: Act on the liver and skeletal muscle, sensitising these tissues to the effects of insulin and consequently increase glucose uptake. These are expensive drugs. They can be used:

1. as a monotherapy, particularly in obese patients, where metformin is contraindicated or not tolerated
2. in combination therapy with metformin or a sulphonylurea, where there is insufficient glycaemic control with one of the former medications alone
3. as part of a triple therapy with metformin and sulphonylurea in patients with insufficient glycaemic control despite dual therapy.

Examples: Pioglitazone, rosiglitazone.

Common and important side effects: Glitazones have been associated with pulmonary oedema, anaemia and distal fractures in female patients. Therefore, they are avoided in patients with evidence of heart failure or those at high risk of fractures.

v. DPP-4 inhibitors (gliptins)

Mechanism of action: Prevent breakdown of incretins released after a meal, therefore increasing insulin secretion and inhibiting pancreatic glucagon release.

Examples: Sitagliptin, vildagliptin.

vi. GLP-1 mimetics

Mechanism of action: GLP-1 is an incretin hormone released by the ileum in a glucose-dependent manner. GLP-1 increases insulin secretion, increases insulin sensitivity, inhibits glucagon release and increases satiety.

Examples: Exenatide.

Insulins

Insulin is a potent and lifesaving medication. Insufficient understanding and errors in prescribing insulin can cause harm to patients.

There are several types of insulin, which all vary with duration of action and time to peak. These are shown below.

Short acting

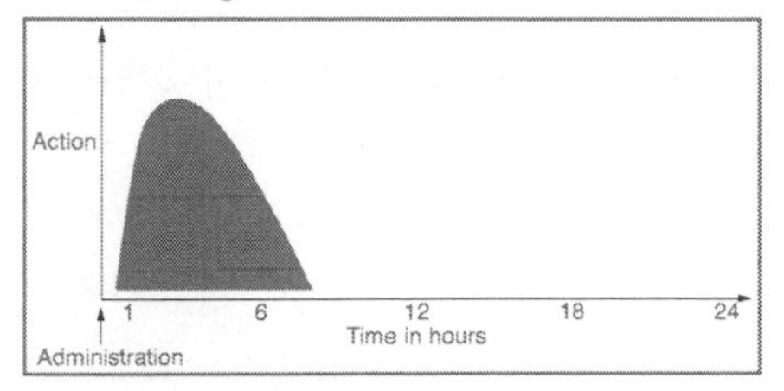

Onset: 30 minutes
Peak: 1–3 hours
Duration: up to 8 hours

Types:
Actrapid, Humulin S

Rapid acting (inject just before meals)

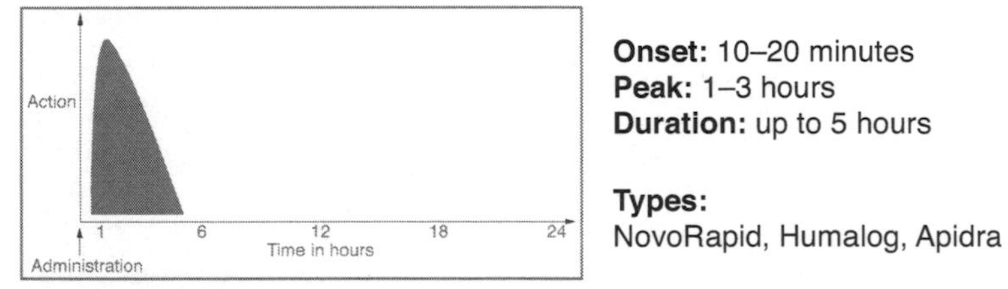

Onset: 10–20 minutes
Peak: 1–3 hours
Duration: up to 5 hours

Types:
NovoRapid, Humalog, Apidra

Intermediate (taken once or twice a day)

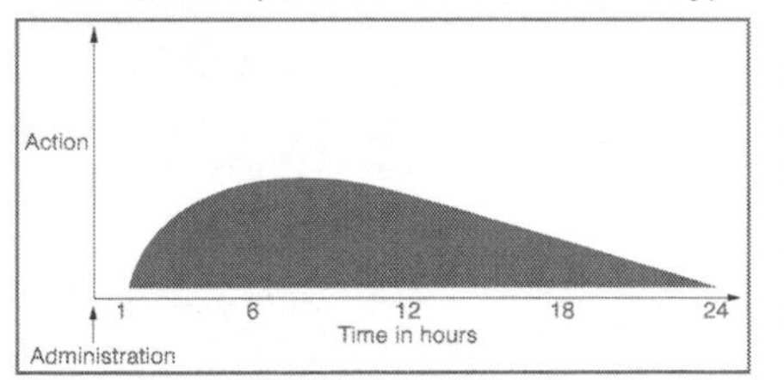

Onset: 90 minutes
Peak: 4–12 hours
Duration: up to 24 hours

Types:
Humulin I

Mixture (taken 20–30 minutes before food)

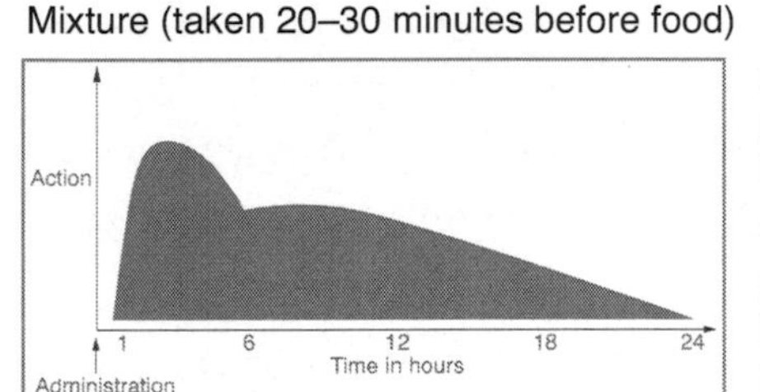

Onset: 30 minutes
Peak: 2–8 hours
Duration: up to 24 hours

Types:
Mixed insulins – Mixtard 30, Humulin M3
Mixed analogues – Humalog Mix 25, Humalog Mix 50, Novomix 30

Mixture (taken once or twice a day, at same time each day)

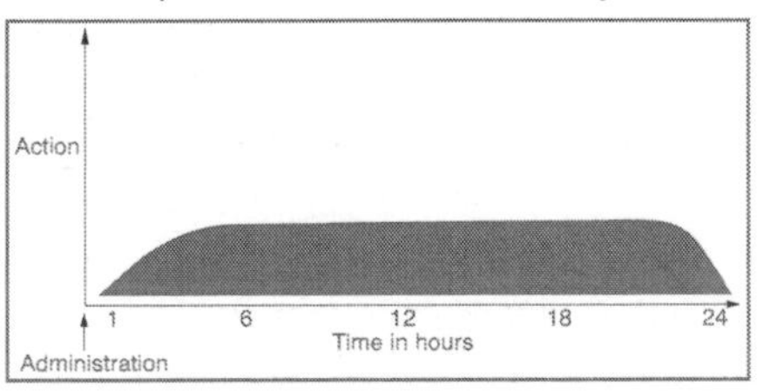

Onset: 24–48 hours
Peak: extended activity
Duration: up to 24 hours

Types:
Long-acting insulin – Insulatard
Long-acting analogue – Lantus, Levemir

Variable rate insulin infusion

Insulin therapy is often the safest and most effective method of gaining glycaemic control in hospital, even in patients not normally treated with insulin. Oral hypoglycaemic agents do not have the flexibility to control the rapidly changing glucose concentration seen in hospital.

Variable rate intravenous infusion of insulin is appropriate in hyperglycaemic diabetic emergencies, pre-operatively for major surgery and when patients are nil-by-mouth. However, insulin has a relatively narrow therapeutic range, which requires careful dose adjustment, administration and monitoring. Also, illness can have unpredictable effects on glycaemic control. Therefore, insulin infusions should be administered with proactive monitoring of blood glucose with appropriate dose adjustment.

Intravenous insulin should be given through a dedicated cannula through which no other medication is administered. Though glycaemic targets should be individualised to the patient, pre-meal glucose concentrations of >5.0 and <7.8 mmol/L and random concentrations <10 mmol/L are suggested.

Indications for variable rate intravenous insulin infusion

- Treating hyperglycaemia when patients are unable to eat or drink, including peri-operative nil-by-mouth status
- Acute illness in diabetic patients for which prompt glycaemic control is important for recovery, e.g. for the prevention or treatment of infection
- Acute illness in non-diabetic patients with secondary hyperglycaemia
- Acute coronary syndrome
- For 48 hours after cardiac surgery

Four steps to prescribing variable rate intravenous insulin infusion

Fast-acting human soluble insulin or an analogue, such as Actrapid, Novorapid or Humulin, is used for intravenous infusion.

Step 1: Insulin infusion

Prescribe the insulin infusion in the 'Infusion Therapy' section of the patient's drug charts.

FLUID	VOLUME	RATE	DRUG ADDED	DOSE
0.9% Sodium chloride	50 mL	Regimen X	Human Soluble Insulin	50 units

Step 2: Insulin rate regimen

Below this, transcribe the variable rate regimens.

BLOOD GLUCOSE (MMOL/L)	INSULIN INFUSION RATE (UNITS/HOUR)			
	REGIMEN A	REGIMEN B	REGIMEN C	REGIMEN D
0–4.0	0 and treat hypo	0 and treat hypo	0 and treat hypo	0 and treat hypo
4.1–6.0	1	1	2	3
6.1–8.0	2	3	4	5
8.1–10.0	3	4	6	8
>10.0	4	6	8	10

Check blood glucose every hour.
If blood glucose >10.0 for 4 hours, move to next higher infusion rate and escalate if high blood glucose persists.

- Patients that are new to insulin should be started with infusion regimen A and titrated to achieve the target blood glucose concentrations.
- Patients already on insulin treatment (exceeding 100 units/24 hours) should be started on regimen B.
- Patients taking long-acting insulin or insulin analogues, such as Lantus or Levemir, should continue to be prescribed these medications, which are to be administered alongside the insulin infusion.

Step 3: Glucose co-infusion

Hypoglycaemia is a potential complication of intensified insulin therapy.

Therefore, intravenous insulin infusions should be supported by glucose or carbohydrate. In most patients, this is by a simultaneous glucose infusion as below.

The rate of the glucose infusion is administered as follows:

- If the patient is unable to eat or drink, start at 125 mL/hour (i.e. 1 L/8 hours).
- If the patient is eating and drinking, start at 80 mL/hour (i.e. 1 L/12 hours).
- If the patient is at risk of fluid overload, start at 30 mL/hour (i.e. 1 L/24 hours).

Prescribe glucose 5% as a co-infusion as below.

FLUID	VOLUME	RATE	DRUG ADDED	DOSE
5% Dextrose	1 L	X mL/hour	–	–

Step 4: Glucose p.r.n. for hypoglycaemia

Hypoglycaemia may develop despite provision of a glucose co-infusion. In addition to the ongoing insulin infusion itself, be aware that the following can also precipitate hypoglycaemia:

- reduced carbohydrate intake
- inappropriate or incorrect prescription or administration of antidiabetic medications
- major amputation of a limb
- severe hepatic dysfunction
- renal dialysis therapy
- impaired renal function
- terminal illness
- food malabsorption including gastroenteritis or coeliac disease
- concurrent use of drugs with hypoglycaemic agents, e.g. warfarin, quinine, salicylates, sulphonamides, MAO-inhibitors, NSAIDs and SSRIs

- loss of anti-insulin hormone function, e.g. Addison's disease, growth hormone deficiency, hypothyroidism, hypopituitarism.

In the 'As required medications' section of the patient's drug chart, prescribe 15–20 g quick-acting carbohydrate to be given every 15 minutes, with repeat blood glucose measurements every 15 minutes. Examples include:

150–200 ml fruit juice

90–120 ml Lucozade Original

4–5 Glucotabs

'Glucogel' 3–4 heaped teaspoons of sugar dissolved in water.

In the acute management of patients who have a hypoglycaemic event while on variable rate intravenous insulin infusion, review the possible causes and consider stepping down to a lower regimen.

In patients who are nil-by-mouth, give 75–80 mL of 20% glucose or 150–160 mL of 10% glucose over 10–15 minutes, via the infusion pump if possible. Check blood glucose levels after 10 minutes and repeat glucose infusion if it is still less than 4 mmol/L.

References

National Health Service Diabetes. *Safe and Effective use of Insulin in Hospitalised Patients*. NHS Diabetes; 2010.

National Institute for Clinical Excellence. *Diagnosis and Management of Type 1 Diabetes in Children, Young People and Adults*: NICE Guideline 15. London: NICE; 2004. www.nice.org.uk/guidance/CG15

National Institute for Clinical Excellence. *Type 2 Diabetes: newer agents (partial update of CG66) (CG87)*: NICE Guideline 87. London: NICE; 2009. www.nice.org.uk/guidance/CG87

National Institute for Clinical Excellence. *Type 2 Diabetes (partially updated by CG87) (CG66)*: NICE Guideline 66. London: NICE; 2008. www.nice.org.uk/guidance/CG66

9

Alcohol withdrawal

Alcohol-related complications include:

- acute withdrawal
- seizures
- delirium tremens (DT)
- Wernicke's encephalopathy
- alcoholic liver disease
- acute and chronic pancreatitis.

An accurate history of the alcohol intake should be documented. Patients should be screened for alcohol dependence and the risk of developing delirium tremens or seizures.

Alcohol withdrawal signs and symptoms

Abrupt cessation or marked reduction of alcohol intake in patients who have drunk excessively over a prolonged period of time can develop a severe, and sometimes fatal, withdrawal syndrome characterised by increased autonomic activity.

Symptoms of withdrawal usually begin within **24 hours** of the last intake of alcohol and peak at 48–72 hours. A drop in blood-alcohol concentration may precipitate a withdrawal syndrome characterised by the following symptoms.

Cognitive and neurological

- Poor concentration
- Agitation
- Aggression
- Insomnia
- Headache
- Seizures

Autonomic

- Tachycardia
- Hypertension
- Tremor
- Sweating
- Nausea
- Vomiting
- Fever

In 5% of patients, this may progress to **delirium tremens (DTs)** characterised by delirium, auditory or visual hallucinations, coarse tremor, disorientation and reduced consciousness. This can be fatal and is a medical emergency requiring senior clinical input. DTs often peak later – at **96 hours** after the patient's last drink.

Investigations should include:

- urea and electrolytes, including magnesium and phosphate
- full blood count
- blood glucose
- liver function tests
- clotting screen
- folate and B_{12}.

Treatment

Treatment should involve:

- benzodiazepine (e.g. chlordiazepoxide)
- nutrition (beware of re-feeding syndrome)
- multivitamins
- thiamine (intravenous and oral)
- fluid and electrolyte replacement
- referral to a drug and alcohol service as appropriate.

Benzodiazepines

These are used to attenuate withdrawal symptoms. Longer acting benzodiazepines offer a smoother withdrawal and provide effective control of withdrawal symptoms within 24–48 hours.

Oral chlordiazepoxide is often the first-line benzodiazepine of choice, although some units may prefer lorazepam or diazepam. If symptoms persist or oral medication is declined, medication can be given parenterally.

Equivalent doses:
Chlordiazepoxide 30 mg = diazepam 10 mg = lorazepam 1 mg.

Benzodiazepine withdrawal regimen

Patients can either be started on a fixed-dose regimen or a more flexible symptom-triggered regimen.

1. A fixed-dose regimen

Benzodiazepine dose is reduced over 5–6 days. P.r.n. doses should be prescribed for breakthrough symptoms. The regime should be reviewed on a daily basis and tailored to individual patient needs.

The following fixed-dose regimen is appropriate for those patients with previous DTs, seizures or moderate alcohol withdrawal. Treatment should be started as soon as the patients can tolerate oral medication and reviewed daily.

DAY	REGULAR DOSE	AS REQUIRED
1	30 mg q.d.s.	10 mg p.r.n. (to a max 200 mg/24 hrs)
2	20 mg q.d.s.	10 mg p.r.n. (to a max 200 mg/24 hrs)
3	20 mg t.d.s.	
4	20 mg b.d.	
5	10 mg b.d.	
6	STOP	

Considerations:

- The dose should be adjusted to provide effective sedative and anticonvulsant endpoints while preventing oversedation, respiratory depression and hypotension.
- Patients may experience seizure as the dose of chlordiazepoxide is tailed off.
- Doses of chlordiazepoxide should be reduced in severe liver dysfunction, the elderly and the frail. Patients with chronic liver disease should have their dose more regularly to avoid over-sedation.
- If more than 3 'p.r.n.' doses are required in 24 hours, reconsider reducing the next day's dose.
- **A maximum of 24 hours (10 mg twice a day) may be prescribed on discharge**. A patient who self-discharges against medical advice must not be prescribed benzodiazepines because taking benzodiazepines while continuing to drink alcohol is dangerous.

2. A symptom-triggered flexible regimen

In severe cases of alcohol withdrawal syndrome (AWS) and on specialist ward areas, a symptom-triggered flexible regimen may be more appropriate. The dose of benzodiazepine is tailored to the patient's requirements as determined by the severity of their withdrawal signs and symptoms.

Patients severely agitated/refractory to benzodiazepines

Achieving early and effective sedation with benzodiazepines is the mainstay of both preventing and treating DTs. However, patients with marked agitation, psychotic symptoms, hallucinations, DTs or at risk of DTs may require antipsychotics as an adjunctive therapy to benzodiazepines. Antipsychotics should not be used alone as they do not treat alcohol withdrawal and may lower the seizure threshold. Wernicke's encephalopathy and hepatic encephalopathy in patients with chronic liver disease should be excluded before starting antipsychotics.

Haloperidol (1–2 mg i.v./i.m. or 1.5–5 mg b.d. p.o.; lower dose in elderly) can be used for marked agitation.

Withdrawal seizures

Seizures usually respond to lorazepam 2 mg i.v. or diazepam 5 mg p.r. repeated after 5 minutes if required. **Phenytoin should *not* be offered to treat alcohol withdrawal seizures.**

Nutrition and vitamin supplementation

Poor nutrition is common in such patients because of inadequate dietary intake, associated chronic liver disease, chronic pancreatitis and malabsorption. Water and fat-soluble vitamins should be replaced and severely malnourished patients should be considered for early enteral feeding via a nasogastric tube. These patients are at risk of developing refeeding syndrome, and may require magnesium, potassium and phosphate supplementation.

Patients with alcohol dependence are at risk of developing **Wernicke's encephalopathy (WE)**, caused by a deficiency in thiamine (vitamin B_1). Patients at most risk are malnourished or have decompensated liver disease. Persistent vomiting can also lead to WE.

WE is characterised by:

- cognitive symptoms: acute confusion, reduced consciousness, amnesia
- ataxia/unsteadiness
- visual symptoms: ophthalmoplegia or nystagmus.

Untreated or inappropriately managed WE will progress to Korsakoff's psychosis characterised by:

- memory loss
- confabulation.

Treatment is with thiamine replacement. WE is initially reversible with high-dose parenteral B vitamins, so treatment should be initiated as soon as possible after a diagnosis is suspected or risk factors identified.

Thiamine

Intravenous thiamine

Oral thiamine is poorly absorbed. Parenteral thiamine (as Pabrinex) should be given as prophylaxis for all patients prescribed a chlordiazepoxide-reducing regimen and/or who have risk factors for WE. This should be given once daily for 3 days or until the patient can take oral thiamine.

Pabrinex i.v.; 2–3 pairs 8 hourly

Oral thiamine

After 3 days of intravenous Pabrinex, thiamine 100 mg p.o. b.d. should be given. Thiamine tablets dispersed in water if administered via a nasogastric tube.

Thiamine 100 mg p.o. b.d.

Other vitamins

In addition to thiamine patients should be prescribed a **multivitamin 1 tablet p.o. o.d.**

Oral multivitamin supplements should be continued in patients who remain malnourished or continue to have inadequate diets. Thiamine should be continued long term if there is cognitive impairment or peripheral neuropathy at a dose of 100 mg b.d. p.o.

Fluid and electrolyte balance

Sedated patients and patients who have a history of alcohol dependence are at risk of dehydration.

- Monitor fluid balance, urea and electrolytes daily.
- Oral intake should be around 2–2.5 L/day in patients *without* decompensated liver disease.
- Potassium, magnesium and phosphate replacement may be required as described above.
- Measure blood glucose daily.

Follow-up

Patients should be provided with information regarding relevant alcohol support and counselling services.

References

National Institute for Clinical Excellence. *Alcohol-use Disorders: physical complications*: NICE Guideline 100. London: NICE; 2010. www.nice.org.uk/guidance/CG100

Scottish Intercollegiate Guidelines Network. *The Management of Harmful Drinking and Alcohol Dependence in Primary Care: a national clinical guideline*. Edinburgh: SIGN; 2003.

10

Prescription charts

The format of these prescription charts consists of a clinical vignette followed by patient pharmacological treatment, in the form of a prescription chart.

The treatment outlined for each patient puts forward the recommended treatment sourced from local or national guidelines, which are correct at the time of publication.

Note that the treatment of the following conditions may be different as based on local policy or changing guidelines.

Good prescribing principles

- Prescribe antimicrobials only when clinically justified and use narrow-spectrum therapy where possible
- Review empirical antimicrobial therapy promptly and change to pathogen-directed therapy or discontinue as appropriate
- Always document the indication and course length or review date of antimicrobials
- Review i.v. antimicrobials at 48 hours and switch to oral if appropriate. Indications include: 1. Afebrile for 48 hours 2. Improving signs/ symptoms 3. Improving clinical markers including falling white cell count and C-reactive Protein 4.

Respiratory

1. Acute asthma

You have been called to see a 21-year-old patient in A&E who has presented with shortness of breath, wheeze and difficulty in completing sentences.

He is a known asthmatic, normally controlled on salbutamol and beclomethasone inhalers. He had recently taken ibuprofen for an injury sustained during a rugby match.

OBSERVATIONS	
Respiratory rate (breaths per minute)	29
Heart rate (beats per minute)	120
Blood pressure (mmHg)	106/63
Oxygen saturation (%)	88% on air
Temperature (°C)	36.7

On examination, he has widespread wheeze and a bounding radial pulse. His peak expiratory flow in A&E was measured as 45% of his best.

You have made a diagnosis of **acute severe exacerbation of asthma**. A chest X-ray excluded rib fractures and pneumothorax. Please complete a prescription chart for this patient.

In adults, severity can be assessed as follows:

SEVERITY	CLINICAL FINDINGS	PEAK EXPIRATORY FLOW (% OF BEST/ESTIMATE)	OTHER MEASUREMENTS
Moderate	No features of severe asthma	50–75	
Acute Severe	RR >25/min HR >110 Inability to complete sentences in 1 breath	33–50	
Life Threatening	Altered consciousness Exhaustion Arrhythmia Hypotension Cyanosis Silent chest Poor respiratory effort	<33	SpO_2 <2% PaO_2 <8 kPa NORMAL $PaCO_2$ (4.6–6 kPa)
Near fatal	As above	–	RAISED $PaCO_2$

In this case, the patient has an acute **severe attack**, which is likely to be due to the use of non-steroidal anti-inflammatory drugs (NSAIDs), which are contraindicated in patients with asthma.

CHART	PRESCRIPTION
Stat.	Salbutamol, 5 mg, Neb Ipratropium bromide, 500 micrograms, Neb. with oxygen Hydrocortisone, 100 mg, i.v.
Oxygen	15 L via non-rebreathing bag, Target saturations 94–98% (continuous)
Regular	Oxygen, 8 L, inh, via non-rebreather mask (Aim for Sats. 94–98%, Repeat ABGs/15 min), All day Salbutamol (oxygen driven), 5 mg, Neb, q.d.s. Ipratropium bromide (oxygen driven), 500 micrograms, Neb, q.d.s.* Hydrocortisone, 100 mg, q.d.s. for 24 hours (omit first dose) Prednisolone, 30 mg, p.o., o.d., 5/7 (omit 1st day) VTE prophylaxis as appropriate
P.R.N.	Salbutamol, 5 mg, Nebs, Max 1 hourly Peak Flow Meter, p.o., q.d.s.
Fluids	None
CI/Stop	Beta-blockers, NSAIDs

* Ipratropium bromide is combined with a nebulised β_2-agonist for significantly greater bronchodilation. It is only indicated in acute severe or life-threatening asthma or those with a poor initial response to β_2-agonist therapy.

Considerations

A single dose of **magnesium sulphate 1.2–2 g i.v.** may be indicated in acute severe, life-threatening or near fatal asthma. However, it should only be used after consultation with seniors.

Intravenous **aminophylline** is not routinely indicated.

Infective exacerbations of asthma are likely to be viral. Routine prescription of **antibiotics** is also not routinely indicated.

Always monitor the patient for response to treatment by regular examination and measurement of peak flow rate. Patients who are failing to respond to therapy and continue to deteriorate, particularly those who have **hypercapnoeic respiratory failure**, will need referral to a high-dependency unit care ± ventilation. Patients who have symptomatic relief and improve should eventually be weaned from oral steroids and initiated on inhaled steroids.

Reference

Scottish Intercollegiate Guidelines Network/British Thoracic Society. *British Guideline on the Management of Asthma*. NHS Quality Improvement Scotland; 2011.

2. Acute COPD exacerbation

You have clerked a 50-year-old patient in A&E. He is a known smoker (25 pack/year history) with a BMI of 32. He has been recently diagnosed with a new condition, for which he has been prescribed Seretide (salmeterol and beclomethasone). He admits to having worsening breathlessness and a productive cough, with thick green sputum.

On examination, he is dyspnoeic, has an inspiratory wheeze and expiratory crepitations across his left middle and lower zones. His symptoms have not responded to salbutamol or Seretide inhalers at home.

OBSERVATIONS	
Respiratory rate (breaths per minute)	29
Heart rate (beats per minute)	120
Blood pressure (mmHg)	106/63
Oxygen saturation (%)	88% on air
Temperature (°C)	36.7
Patient has systemic inflammatory response syndrome (SIRS)	

A chest X-ray and ECG have been requested; sputum has been collected for microscopy and culture, and blood cultures have been sent before commencing empirical antibiotic treatment.

The registrar has asked you to complete a drug chart on the basis that he has an **infective exacerbation of COPD.** In the presence of clinical and radiological pneumonia in known COPD, this is the most likely diagnosis; however, consider differentials including pulmonary embolism, left heart failure, and arrhythmias.

Severity of COPD can be judged as follows.

POST-BRONCHODILATOR FEV1/FVC	FEV1 % OF PREDICTED	SEVERITY
<0.7	>80%	Mild
<0.7	50–79%	Moderate
<0.7	30–49%	Severe
<0.7	<30%	Very severe

SIRS = Temperature >38 or <36 | Heart rate >90 | Respiratory rate >20 or $PaCO_2$ <4.3 kPa | WBC <4 or >12 × 10^9/L.

Sepsis = SIRS in the presence of infection.

Severe sepsis = Sepsis with organ dysfunction.

Septic shock = Severe sepsis with systolic blood pressure <90 mmHg despite adequate resuscitation.

Management of sepsis initially entails empiric treatment as outlined in the national *Surviving Sepsis* guidelines.

CHART	PRESCRIPTION
Stat.	Salbutamol, 5 mg, Neb Ipratropium bromide, 500 micrograms, Neb Hydrocortisone, 100 mg, i.v. Co-amoxiclav, 625 mg, p.o.
Oxygen	4 L/min via Venturi mask (FiO_2 28%), Target saturations 88–92% (continuous) Titrate appropriately*
Regular	Salbutamol (air driven), 2.5 mg, Neb, 4-hourly Ipratropium bromide (air driven), 500 micrograms, Neb, q.d.s. Prednisolone, 30 mg, p.o., o.d. 7/7 (omit 1st day) Co-amoxiclav, 625 mg, p.o., t.d.s. (5/7, omit 1st dose) Paracetamol, 1 g, p.o., q.d.s. Carbocisteine, 75 mg, p.o., t.d.s. VTE prophylaxis as appropriate
P.R.N.	Salbutamol, 5 mg, Nebs, Max q.d.s.
Fluids	
CI/Stop	

* Acutely unwell and rapidly deteriorating patients should receive high-flow oxygen aiming for saturations of 94%–98% via non-rebreathing bag. If they are at risk of hypercapnic respiratory failure (type 2 respiratory failure) start 24% (2 L) or 28% (4 L) oxygen via Venturi mask, aiming for saturations of 88%–92%.

Patients should be monitored with pulse oximetry and regular arterial blood gas measurements to guide further oxygen titration and hypercapnic respiratory failure. Deteriorating patients may be candidates for NIV (e.g. BiPAP) or ITU admission.

A patient suffering from COPD is susceptible to infective exacerbations, especially during the winter. Those who have an increase in breathlessness and sputum purulence should be treated with an antibiotic. The choice of antibiotic is dependent upon local and trust guidelines – an aminopenicillin, a macrolide (e.g. azithromycin) or a tetracycline (e.g. doxycycline) should be prescribed. In this case a 5-day course of co-amoxiclav has been prescribed. In patients with severe sepsis, this can be given i.v. (1.2 g t.d.s.). Note that doxycycline is contraindicated in pregnancy.

Reference

National Institute for Clinical Excellence. *Chronic Obstructive Pulmonary Disease: management of chronic obstructive pulmonary disease in adults in primary and secondary care (partial update)*: NICE Guideline 101. London: NICE; 2010. www.nice.org.uk/guidance/CG101

3. Moderate pneumonia

You see a 69-year-old Greek homeless man in the emergency department. He has been living intermittently on the street and in shelters, and it has been a particularly difficult and cold month. The patient is a non-smoker and has no history of exposure to tuberculosis, and no weight loss or night sweats.

He appears short of breath, and while talking to him it is evident that he has a productive cough, with thick green sputum. History reveals a 3-day history of fevers, rigors, malaise and cough, with occasional bouts of pleuritic chest pain.

OBSERVATIONS	
Respiratory rate (breaths per minute)	27
Heart rate (beats per minute)	100
Blood pressure (mmHg)	110/81
Oxygen saturation (%)	93% on air
Temperature (°C)	38.2

Upon listening to his chest, there is decreased air entry to the left lower zone, which is also dull to percussion. Chest X-ray confirms a defined consolidation in the left lower zone.

Bloods reveal Urea 8 mmol/L, white cell count 12×10^9/L, CRP 42 mg/L and normal liver function tests and electrolytes. You send a sample of sputum for microscopy, culture and PCR, bloods for microscopy and culture, and a sample of urine for *Legionella* and *Pneumococcus* antigen tests. It is likely that this patient is suffering from a community-acquired pneumonia (CAP), CURB^{65} Score of 2 indicating moderate severity. Please write up a drug chart to manage the infection.

Severity of CAP is measured by the CURB^{65} score:

C – Confusion (MTS <8 or new disorientation in person/place/time)
U – Urea >7 mmol/L
R – Respiratory rate >30/min
B – Blood pressure (systolic <90 or diastolic <60)
65 – Age >65

CURB[65] Score of 0: Low severity CAP – oral antibiotics in the community.

CURB[65] Score of 2: Moderate risk of death – consider short-stay inpatient therapy with amoxicillin and a macrolide as soon as possible.

CURB[65] Score of 3 or more: High risk of death – assess with consideration for transfer to critical care unit.

CHART	PRESCRIPTION
Stat.	Amoxicillin, 500 mg, p.o. Clarithromycin, 500 mg, p.o. Paracetamol, 1 g, p.o./i.v.
Oxygen	15 L via non-rebreathing bag, Target saturations 94–98% (continuous)
Regular	Amoxicillin, 500 mg, p.o./i.v., t.d.s. for 7/7 (omit 1st dose) Clarithromycin, 500 mg, p.o./i.v., b.d. for 7/7 (omit 1st dose) Paracetamol, 1 g, p.o., q.d.s. VTE prophylaxis as appropriate
P.R.N.	
Fluids	0.9% saline, 1 L, 20 mmol KCL over 4 hrs* Dextrose 5%, 1 L, 20 mmol KCL over 6 hrs* Dextrose 5%, 1 L, 20 mmol KCL over 8 hrs*
CI/Stop	Use ceftriaxone, 2 g, i.v., o.d. in patients who are allergic to penicillin or macrolides. Use intravenous amoxicillin/benzylpenicillin in combination with clarithromycin where oral therapy is contraindicated.

* Monitor K^+ and urea to guide fluid resuscitation.

Reference

British Thoracic Society. *BTS Guidelines for the Management of Community Acquired Pneumonia in Adults*. British Thoracic Society; 2010.

4. Severe pneumonia

You see an 89-year-old female patient brought into A&E from a nursing home with a 2-day history of a productive cough and high fever. She is known to have a good cognitive baseline but has become increasingly confused over the last 12 hours.

On admission her GCS is 10/15 and her basic observations are as follows.

OBSERVATIONS	
Respiratory rate (breaths per minute)	31
Heart rate (beats per minute)	92
Blood pressure (mmHg)	86/42
Oxygen saturation (%)	Unrecordable
Temperature (°C)	35.1

You assess and manage her treatment using the ABCDE approach. Blood and urine are sent for appropriate investigations as previously discussed (Scenario 3) and she has a portable chest X-ray.

She has a CURB^{65} score (preceding blood analysis) of 4 and is in septic shock. She is diagnosed with severe community-acquired pneumonia, which is associated with a high mortality rate.

CHART	PRESCRIPTION
Stat.	Paracetamol, 1 g, p.o./i.v. Co-amoxiclav, 1.2 g, i.v. Clarithromycin, 500 mg, i.v. Gelofusin, 500 ml, i.v.
Oxygen	15 L via non-rebreathe bag, Target saturations 94–98% (continuous)
Regular	Co-amoxiclav, 1.2 g, i.v., t.d.s. for 7/7 Clarithromycin, 500 mg, i.v., b.d. for 7/7 Paracetamol, 1 g, i.v./p.o. q.d.s. VTE prophylaxis as appropriate
P.R.N.	
Fluids	0.9% Saline, 1 L, 20 mmol KCL over 4 hrs Dextrose 5%, 1 L, 20 mmol KCL over 6 hrs Dextrose 5%, 1 L, 20 mmol KCL over 8 hrs
CI/Stop	Give a second- (Cefuroxime) or third-generation (Cefotaxime/ Ceftriaxone) cephalosporin to patients who are penicillin-allergic, instead of co-amoxiclav. Consider levofloxacin if *Legionella* is strongly suspected.

Cardiovascular

5. ST segment elevated myocardial infarction (STEMI)

A 61-year-old investment banker has attended A&E with acute onset sudden chest pain. The pain is central and crushing in nature, radiating to his left arm and jaw, with a score of 8/10. The pain has been continuous for 30 minutes with no improvement. He suffers from hypercholesterolaemia and takes atorvastatin 20 mg nocte. A 12-lead ECG shows the following.

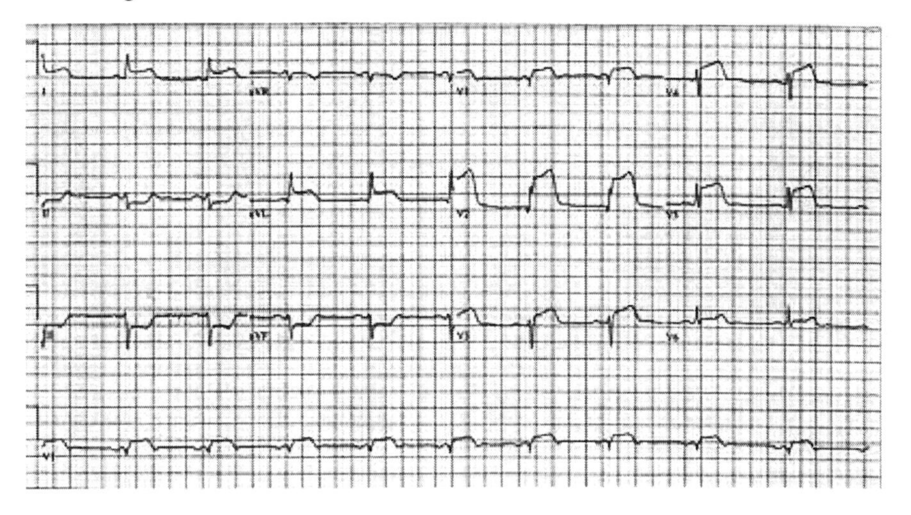

This patient has an acute coronary syndrome – specifically an ST-elevated myocardial infarction (STEMI). Patients suffering from a STEMI have myocardial necrosis. A specialty doctor should decide between early thrombolysis or percutaneous intervention (PCI). ECG evidence of a STEMI may include one or more of the following: i) a 1 mm rise in 2 or more limb leads or ii) a 2 mm rise in 2 or more consecutive chest leads or iii) new Left Bundle Branch Block or iv) a posterior infarction. Note 20% of ECGs will be initially normal. Continuous cardiac rhythm monitoring has been commenced and bloods have been sent for analysis (including troponin, glucose and cholesterol). You have been asked to write a prescription chart for the patient.

CHART	PRESCRIPTION
Stat.	Morphine sulphate IR, 5–10 mg, i.v. Metoclopramide, 10 mg, i.v. Glyceryl trinitrate, 2 puffs, s.l. Aspirin, 300 mg, p.o. Clopidogrel, 600 mg, p.o. Atenolol, 5 mg, i.v. over 5 min (unless hypotensive or bradycardic) Lower molecular weight Heparin, e.g. Enoxaparin, 30 mg, i.v.
Oxygen	15 L via non-rebreathing bag, Target saturations 94–98% (continuous)
Regular	Aspirin, 75 mg, p.o., o.d. Ramipril, 2.5 mg, p.o., b.d. (start 3 days after MI!) Bisoprolol, 5 mg, p.o., o.d. Atorvastatin, 20 mg, p.o., nocte. Clopidogrel, 75 mg, p.o., o.d. (for 1 year) LMWH, e.g. Enoxaparin, 1 mg/kg, s.c., b.d. (8 days) TEDS, 2 tabs, top, All day circle
P.R.N.	Paracetamol, 1 g, p.o./i.v., q.d.s. Morphine sulphate IR, 5–10 mg, p.o./i.m./i.v./, Max 4-hrly Metoclopramide, 10 mg, i.v./i.m., Max t.d.s. Lactulose, 10 mL, p.o., Max b.d. (for constipation) Glyceryl trinitrate, 2 puffs, s.l., Max 2 hrs (for chest pain)
Fluids	**Consider GTN infusion if evidence of LVF:** Normal saline, 50 mL, 50 mg glyceryl trinitrate, Rate 10 mL/hr (titrate to pain, stop if SBP <100)
CI/Stop	Clopidogrel only in Aspirin allergy

In patients with an acute coronary syndrome and diabetes mellitus or marked hyperglycaemia (BM >11.0 mmol/L), begin immediate intensive blood glucose control for at least 24 hours.

Reference

Scottish Intercollegiate Guidelines Network. *Acute Coronary Syndromes: a national clinical guideline*. SIGN Guideline 93; 2010.

6. Non-ST segment elevated myocardial infarction (NSTEMI)

A 70-year-old publican attends A&E complaining of a central crushing chest pain radiating to his jaw, which began 20 minutes ago. The patient complains of nausea, though he has not vomited, and he is sweating, anxious and short of breath. His pain has not responded to three courses of his GTN spray.

The patient has a history of ischaemic heart disease, left ventricular failure and eczema. He has a 30 pack/year history of smoking and drinks approximately 22 units of alcohol each week.

OBSERVATIONS	
Respiratory rate (breaths per minute)	22
Heart rate (beats per minute)	130
Blood pressure (mmHg)	113/72
Oxygen saturation (%)	94% on air
Temperature (°C)	36.8

He is placed on cardiac monitoring. A troponin-T test (normal range 0–0.04) shows a level of 1.1 ng/mL at 2 hours. An ECG confirms LVF, but no evidence of ST-elevation. In a patient presenting with this history it is suggestive of a non-ST elevation myocardial infarction.

All patients should be assessed for risk with an established risk scoring system that predicts 6-month mortality, such as Global Registry of Acute Cardiac Events (GRACE). This patient has a high 6-month mortality risk. A specialty doctor should decide whether to use a GPI (Tirofiban or eptifibatide), whether angiography is indicated. Fondaparinus is indicated in patients unless there is a high bleeding risk or angiography is planned within 24 hours.

Write a prescription chart to manage the NSTEMI in the acute setting.

CHART	PRESCRIPTION
Stat.	Morphine sulphate IR, 5–10 mg, i.v. Metoclopramide, 10 mg, i.v. Glyceryl trinitrate, 2 puffs, s.l. Aspirin, 300 mg, p.o.* Clopidogrel, 300 mg, p.o.* Fondaparinux, 2.5 mg, s.c.*
Oxygen	15 L via non-rebreathing bag, Target saturations 94–98% (continuous)
Regular	Fondaparinux, 2.5 mg, s.c., o.d. (unless PCI within 24 hours) Aspirin, 75 mg, p.o., o.d. Clopidogrel, 75 mg, p.o., o.d. Ramipril, 2.5 mg, p.o., b.d. (start 3 days after MI) Bisoprolol, 5.0 mg, p.o., o.d. Atorvastatin, 20 mg, p.o., nocte. Paracetamol, 1 g, p.o., q.d.s. TEDS, 2 tabs, Top, All day circle
P.R.N.	Morphine sulphate IR, 5–10 mg, p.o./i.v., Max 4-hrly Metoclopramide, 10 mg, i.v./i.m., Max t.d.s. Lactulose, 10 mL, p.o., Max b.d. (for constipation) Glyceryl trinitrate, 2 puffs, s.l., Max 2 hrs (for chest pain)
Fluids	**Given diagnosis of LVF:** Normal saline, 50 mL, 50 mg glyceryl trinitrate, Rate 10 mL/hr (titrate to pain, stop if SBP <100)
CI/Stop	

* Avoid if risk or recent history of bleeding.

- Strictly control blood sugars at <10 mmol/L and consider starting continuous insulin therapy if >10 mmol/L.
- Ramipril reduces ventricular remodelling.
- GP IIa/IIIb inhibitors such as tirofiban are reserved for high-risk patients with ischaemia and elevated troponin.

Reference

Scottish Intercollegiate Guidelines Network. *Acute Coronary Syndromes: a national clinical guideline*. SIGN Guideline 93; 2010.

7. Acute left ventricular failure

A 74-year-old woman was brought in by ambulance to the emergency department with severe shortness of breath and anxiousness. She has a history of rheumatic fever and chronic mitral regurgitation and has been recently started on a beta-blocker for hypertension.

OBSERVATIONS	
Respiratory rate (breaths per minute)	25
Heart rate (beats per minute)	68
Blood pressure (mmHg)	108/62
Oxygen saturation (%)	89%
Temperature (°C)	36.1

On examination she has a raised JVP. Upon auscultation you find a gallop rhythm superimposed on a pansystolic murmur, a laterally displaced apex beat and coarse widespread inspiratory crepitations. She has bilateral pitting oedema to the ankles.

The patient's chest X-ray shows bilateral pulmonary oedema, cardiomegaly and evidence of upper lobe diversion. Her ECG shows evidence of left ventricular hypertrophy but no significant ST-segment changes. Her troponin is not elevated.

After consultation with the medical registrar, your primary diagnosis is acute left ventricular failure, secondary to decompensated mitral regurgitation.

Please complete the drug chart for the patient.

CHART	PRESCRIPTION
Stat.	Diamorphine, 5 mg, i.v. slowly GTN, 2 puffs, s.l. Metoclopramide, 10 mg, i.v. Furosemide, 40 mg, i.v.
Oxygen	15 L via non-rebreathing bag, Target saturations 94–98% (continuous)
Regular	Furosemide, 40 mg, p.o., o.d. VTE prophylaxis as appropriate
P.R.N.	GTN, 2 puffs (400 micrograms), s.l., every 5–10 min
Fluids	If systolic >110 mmHg: Nitroglycerin infusion, 10–20 micrograms/min with regular BP monitoring
CI/Stop	STOP patient's beta-blocker for now

Beta-blockers and ACE-inhibitors reduce the risk of mortality in patients with heart failure. Once the patient has overcome the acute ventricular failure, consider starting long term an ACE-I and beta-blocker.

Reference

European Society of Cardiology. ESC Guidelines for the diagnosis and treatment of acute and chronic heart failure. *Eur Heart J.* 2008; **29**: 2388–442.

Urinary system

8. Urinary tract infection

You have been bleeped by a nurse on your ward to see a 72-year-old patient who is day 5 post-hip hemiarthroplasty. She is now complaining of frequency and dysuria with suprapubic pain, and has a low-grade fever. Her catheter was removed 3 days ago. The nurse has dipsticked the urine and the results are as follows.

MARKER	RESULT
Blood	+
Leucocytes	++
Nitrite	++
Ketone	Trace
Glucose	–
pH	6.5
Urobilinogen	–

She is clinically stable and does not have any signs suggestive of sepsis, so you make a diagnosis of **hospital acquired UTI**. You have asked the nurse to send the urine for microscopy and culture. She is on analgesia for her hip surgery and some hypertensive medication. She is eating and drinking.

Please write her drug chart, together with any other medication she is taking.

CHART	PRESCRIPTION
Stat.	Nitrofurantoin, 50 mg, p.o. OR Co-amoxiclav 625 mg p.o.
Regular	Nitrofurantoin, 50 mg, p.o., q.d.s. 3/7 OR Co-amoxiclav 625 mg p.o., t.d.s. 3/7 Paracetamol, 1 g, p.o., q.d.s. Amlodipine 10 mg, p.o., o.m. VTE prophylaxis as appropriate
P.R.N.	Codeine phosphate, 30 mg, p.o., q.d.s.
Fluids	
CI/Stop	

Considerations

- Encourage good fluid intake (>3 L/day) to maintain diuresis.
- Relapsing infections may need increased doses and treatment for 6–12 months.

A 7-day course of antibiotics is recommended in male patients and all patients who are catheterised and symptomatic.

Avoid nitrofurantoin in patients with renal failure (if eGFR less than 60 mL/minute/1.73 m^2). Avoid co-amoxiclav in patients who are allergic to penicillin. In these circumstances prescribe trimethoprim, 200 mg p.o., b.d.

Reference

Scottish Intercollegiate Guidelines Network. *Management of Suspected Bacterial Urinary Tract Infections in Adults: a national clinical guideline.* SIGN Guideline 88; 2006.

9. Urosepsis/pyelonephritis

You are bleeped by a nurse on the ward to see the same patient in **Scenario 8**. It has been 24 hours since you prescribed her an antibiotic for a hospital acquired UTI, but she has worsened since then. She has vomited three times, and is complaining of rigors and loin pain. She feels clammy and thirsty but cannot hold anything down. She appears clinically dry. She has not passed any urine for 3 hours despite targeted fluid resuscitation.

OBSERVATIONS	
Respiratory rate (breaths per minute)	26
Heart rate (beats per minute)	127
Blood pressure (mmHg)	102/70
Oxygen saturation (%)	96% on air
Temperature (°C)	39.2

This patient has severe sepsis (specifically, systemic inflammatory response syndrome in the presence of infection with evidence of acute kidney injury). You would approach this patient using the ABCDE approach and your initial aim would be fluid resuscitation.

You bleep the medical registrar, who advises you to follow the trust guidelines for urosepsis until they arrive. You send away a sample of urine for microscopy and culture, and treat the infection with empirical antibiotics.

CHART	PRESCRIPTION
Stat.	Gelofusine, 500 mL, i.v. Co-amoxiclav, 1.2 g, i.v. Paracetamol, 1 g, p.o. Cyclizine, 50 mg, p.o.
Oxygen	15 L via non-rebreathing bag, Target saturations 94–98% (continuous)
Regular	Co-amoxiclav, 1.2 g, i.v., t.d.s., 14/7 (omit 1st day dose)* Paracetamol, 1 g, p.o., q.d.s. VTE prophylaxis as appropriate
P.R.N.	Codeine phosphate, 30 mg, p.o., q.d.s. Cyclizine, 50 mg, p.o., t.d.s. Lactulose, 10 mL, p.o., Max b.d. (for constipation)
Fluids	0.9% saline, 1 L, over 4 hrs** Dextrose 5%, 1 L, over 6 hrs** Dextrose 5%, 1 L, 20 mmol KCL over 8 hrs**
CI/Stop	STOP: Antihypertensive medications

* Consider adding gentamicin, 5 mg/kg, i.v.

** Monitor K^+.

Reference

King's College Hospital. *King's College Hospital Adult Inpatient Pocket Antimicrobial Guide*. King's College London NHS Foundation Trust; 2011.

10. Renal colic

You see a 48-year-old male on an orthopaedic ward who has had surgery on his shoulder 6 hours ago. He arrived to the ward 2 days ago for his procedure but it was cancelled on the day and was rescheduled.

He is now complaining of severe colicky pain, which radiates from loin to groin and comes in waves. He complains of strangury since his earlier procedure. He has vomited twice since his procedure and cannot lie still due to the pain.

You dipstick his urine prior to sending it for microscopy and culture.

MARKER	RESULT
Blood	++
Leucocytes	+
Nitrite	+
Ketone	Trace
Glucose	–
pH	7.2
Urobilinogen	–

OBSERVATIONS	
Respiratory rate (breaths per minute)	21
Heart rate (beats per minute)	92
Blood pressure (mmHg)	136/73
Oxygen saturation (%)	98%
Temperature (°C)	37.2

You initially prescribe paracetamol and request a non-contrast helical CT Kidney-Ureters-Bladder (CT KUB). There is 6 mm focal calcification within the proximal left ureter.

The patient has a ureteric calculus but no evidence of sepsis, and no history of kidney disease. At 6 mm, the stone is unlikely to pass with medical management alone. You request review by the on-call urology registrar who agrees to see the patient and take over his care. In the meantime, write up his medication.

CHART	PRESCRIPTION
Stat.	Diclofenac, 75 mg, i.v./i.m. Cyclizine, 50 mg, p.o./i.v.
Oxygen	2 L via nasal cannula, Target saturations 94–98% (p.r.n.)
Regular	Diclofenac 75 mg, p.o., t.d.s. Tamsulosin 400 micrograms, p.o., o.d.* Paracetamol, 1 g, p.o., q.d.s. VTE prophylaxis as appropriate
P.R.N.	Morphine sulphate IR, 2.5–5 mg, p.o./i.v., Max 4-hrly Cyclizine, 50 mg, p.o./i.v., Max t.d.s. Lactulose, 10 mL, p.o., Max b.d. (for constipation)
Fluids	0.9% saline, 1 L, 20 mmol KCL over 8 hrs Dextrose 5%, 1 L, 20 mmol KCL over 8 hrs Dextrose 5%, 1 L, 20 mmol KCL over 8 hrs
CI/Stop	If infective, treat as pyelonephritis/urosepsis STOP OTHER NSAIDs

* Tamsulosin encourages expulsion and reduces the need for analgesics.

Reference

The British Association of Urological Surgeons. *Guidelines for Acute Management of First Presentation of Renal/Ureteric Lithiasis*. The British Association of Urological Surgeons – Section of Endourology; 2008.

Neurology

11. Meningitis

A 16-year-old Bajan female arrives in A&E with a severe headache, neck stiffness and photophobia. She has become increasingly drowsy and has developed a petechial, non-blanching rash across her arms and shoulders. She is otherwise fit and well and has no recent travel history of note.

OBSERVATIONS	
Respiratory rate (breaths per minute)	20
Heart rate (beats per minute)	89
Blood pressure (mmHg)	112/67
Oxygen saturation (%)	96%
Temperature (°C)	37.8

Kernig's sign is positive, and there is bilateral optic disc swelling on fundoscopy. A suspected diagnosis of meningococcal meningitis is made. Antibiotics should be started prior to further investigation. You assess and manage her treatment using the ABCDE approach. Write up the prescription chart for initial therapy of bacterial meningitis, pending blood microscopy and cultures with CSF analysis.

You then arrange for an urgent CT given evidence of reduced consciousness.

CHART	PRESCRIPTION
Stat.	Ceftriaxone, 2 g, i.v. Dexamethasone phosphate, 0.15 mg/kg, i.v.
Oxygen	15 L via non-rebreathing bag, Target saturations 94–98% (PRN)
Regular	Oxygen, 15 L, inh, via non-rebreather mask Dexamethasone phosphate, 0.15 mg/kg, i.v., q.d.s. (omit 1st dose), 4/7 Ceftriaxone, 2 g, i.v., b.d. 10/7 (omit first day) VTE prophylaxis
P.R.N.	
Fluids	0.9% saline, 1 L, 20 mmol KCL over 12 hrs Dextrose 5%, 1 L, 20 mmol KCL over 12 hrs
CI/Stop	CI: **If septicaemic (rash and shock)** do not give dexamethasone If penicillin allergic: chloramphenicol, 25 mg/kg, i.v., q.d.s. + vancomycin i.v. 2/52

If encephalitis suspected add acyclovir, 10 mg/kg, i.v., t.d.s.

If patient is immunocompromised, over 50 years old or *Listeria* is suspected, add amoxicillin, 2 g, i.v., 4-hourly.

Remember to offer prophylaxis to close contacts of patients with meningitis, usually with rifampicin or ciprofloxacin or ceftriaxone.

Reference

National Institute for Clinical Excellence. *Bacterial Meningitis and Meningococcal Septicaemia: management of bacterial meningitis and meningococcal septicaemia in children and young people younger than 16 years in primary and secondary care*: NICE Guideline 102. London: NICE; 2010. www.nice.org.uk/guidance/CG102

12. Seizure

You are a foundation doctor on a busy stroke ward. A nurse who is attending a patient who has had a stroke 4 hours ago has put out an emergency call. You hurry to the scene and see that the patient is having a tonic-clonic seizure, which the nurse informs you had started a minute ago.

You immediately adopt the ABCDE approach, and tend to the patient's airway. You ask the nurse to insert an oropharyngeal or nasopharyngeal airway and begin high-flow oxygen via a non-rebreathing bag. The patient has no intravenous access as her cannula was dislodged during the event.

Give **Diazepam Rectubes p.r. 0.5 mg/kg.**

The seizures terminate moments after. O_2 saturations remained above 92% throughout. You cannulate the patient, and shortly afterwards she has another seizure.

Give **Lorazepam 2–4 mg i.v. over 30 seconds.**

Your seniors have arrived as soon as the second seizure ends. In order to prevent another seizure you have been asked to prescribe a loading dose of phenytoin.

Start **Phenytoin 18 mg/kg i.v. infusion, not exceeding rate of 50 mg/min.**

This requires BP and heart rate monitoring.

Throughout the event, you must attempt to ascertain the cause of the seizures. The above patient has had a stroke. Taking blood for FBC, U&E, LFT and glucose will aid further management. If seizures persist or if status epilepticus continues, the patient will require general anaesthesia and admission to ITU.

Reference

Scottish Intercollegiate Guidelines Network. *Diagnosis and Management of Epilepsy in Adults: a national clinical guideline.* SIGN Guideline 70; 2003.

Gastroenterology

13. Management of *Clostridium difficile*

A patient on the respiratory ward who was successfully treated for pneumonia has now developed crampy abdominal pain with Bristol stool chart type 7 diarrhoea. She has a temperature of 38.1 degrees and a white cell count of 12.2×10^9/L. She has been unable to eat and drink since last night and appears clinically dehydrated. The staff nurse has sent a stool sample, which later confirms a positive *C. difficile* toxin. You have been asked by the registrar to write up a prescription chart.

The patient had already been moved to an isolated side room, and barrier nursing commenced, with gloves and apron worn during any patient contact.

Treatment of Clostridium difficile

Mild:

Oral metronidazole 400 mg t.d.s. for 10–14 days

Severe (white cell count >15 × 10^9/L; serum creatinine >50% baseline; temp >38.5 degrees; clinical or radiological evidence of severe *C. difficile*) OR refractory to oral metronidazole:

Oral vancomycin 125 mg q.d.s. for 10–14 days

CHART	PRESCRIPTION
Stat.	Metronidazole, 400 mg, p.o.
Oxygen	
Regular	Metronidazole, 400 mg, p.o., t.d.s., 10/7 (omit 1st dose) VTE prophylaxis as appropriate
P.R.N.	Paracetamol, 1 g, p.o., q.d.s.
Fluids	0.9% saline, 1 L, 20 mmol KCL over 4 hrs Dextrose 5%, 1 L, 20 mmol KCL over 6 hrs Dextrose 5%, 1 L, 20 mmol KCL over 8 hrs
Stop	Stop the offending antibiotic. If this is not possible due to concurrent systemic infection, attempt to use an antibiotic with a low theoretical risk of causing *C. difficile*.

References

Health Protection Network. *Guidance on Prevention and Control of Clostridium difficile Infection (CDI) in Healthcare Settings in Scotland NHS*. National Services Scotland; 2009.

King's College Hospital. *King's College Hospital Adult Inpatient Pocket Antimicrobial Guide*. King's College London NHS Foundation Trust; 2011.

14. Post-operative laparoscopic cholecystectomy

A 66-year-old carpenter has been admitted for an elective laparoscopic cholecystectomy, which will be performed the following morning. You have performed a pre-operative assessment and note that he has Type 2 diabetes, hypertension and persistent AF (rate controlled) for which he takes medication (current INR 1.4).

He has not taken warfarin for 6 days, as advised by the anaesthetist. Please complete a prescription chart for his stay, bearing in mind his current medication (amlodipine 5 mg and digoxin 125 micrograms).

Management of perioperative anticoagulation

Warfarin should be stopped 6 days prior to major surgery. On the day before surgery, INR must be <1.5. If >1.8, vitamin K 1–2 mg p.o./s.c. can be given.

Warfarin should be restarted post-operatively. If it is a procedure with a mild to moderate risk of bleeding (e.g. abdominal surgery as above), it can be restarted at 8 p.m. on the day of the procedure. For procedures with high risk of post-operative bleeding (e.g. vascular surgery or prostatectomy), it should be restarted at 8 p.m. the following day.

The patient has a low risk of thromboembolism (rate-controlled AF), and so can be prescribed thromboprophylaxis on the previous evening and on the day of his procedure.

In patients with a high risk of post-operative thromboembolism, e.g. mechanical heart valve, previous thromboembolic event, known thrombophilia, a *treatment dose* of LMWH should be considered until appropriate post-operative anticoagulation.

CHART	PRESCRIPTION
Stat.	
Oxygen	
Regular	Warfarin, 5 mg, p.o., o.d. (8 p.m. on the day of procedure) Amlodipine, 5 mg, p.o., o.d. Digoxin, 125 micrograms, p.o., o.d. Paracetamol, 1 g, p.o., q.d.s. VTE prophylaxis as appropriate
P.R.N.	Codeine phosphate 30–60 mg p.o., q.d.s. Cyclizine 50 mg p.o./i.v., t.d.s. Lactulose, 10 mL, p.o., max b.d. (for constipation)
Fluids	Hartmann's, 1 L, over 8 hrs

Reference

Royal United Hospital Bath NHS Trust. *Guidelines for the Perioperative Management of Anticoagulation*. Royal United Hospital Bath NHS Trust; 2006.

Dermatology

15. Cellulitis

A 62-year-old woman has been referred to A&E from her GP complaining of a hot, painful and red right shin. She denies any trauma to the area and has noticed a reddening of the skin, which has been expanding over a few days.

On examination her observations are stable and she is apyrexial. The patient's right leg is tender to palpation from the ankle to the mid-shin. She has evidence of bilateral chronic venous insufficiency.

An X-ray of the ankle confirms no bony abnormality. You suspect that the patient has cellulitis. The patient is on metformin (500 mg t.d.s.), for Type 2 diabetes, which she says is normally well controlled. She has no allergies. Please write a drug chart for the patient.

Cellulitis classification (CREST criteria)

	SYMPTOMS	1ST LINE TREATMENT	2ND LINE TREATMENT
Class 1	No systemic signs	Flucloxacillin 500 mg p.o., q.d.s.	Clarithromycin 500 mg p.o., b.d.
Class 2	A patient with a significant comorbidity (e.g. venous ulcer disease, peripheral vascular disease or morbid obesity), with or without systemic signs	Flucloxacillin 2 g i.v., q.d.s.	Clarithromycin 500 mg i.v., b.d.
Class 3	Systemic signs: tachycardia, tachypnoea, hypotension, confusion, low urine output	Flucloxacillin 2 g i.v., q.d.s.	Clarithromycin 500 mg i.v., b.d.
Class 4	Cellulitis complicated by sepsis syndrome or necrotising fasciitis	Benzylpenicillin 2.4 g i.v., 2–4 hourly AND Ciprofloxacin 400 mg i.v., b.d. AND Clindamycin 900 mg i.v., t.d.s.	

This patient is treated as having Class 2 cellulitis.

CHART	PRESCRIPTION
Stat.	Paracetamol, 1 g, p.o.
Oxygen	
Regular	Flucloxacillin 2 g, i.v., q.d.s., review after 7/7 Paracetamol, 1 g, p.o., q.d.s. (omit first dose) Metformin 500 mg t.d.s. VTE prophylaxis as appropriate – do not apply TEDS to the affected leg
P.R.N.	Paracetamol, 1 g, p.o., q.d.s.
Fluids	
Stop	

Reference

Clinical Resource Efficiency Support Team. *Guidelines on the Management of Cellulitis in Adults*. CREST; 2005.

Rheumatology

16. Gout

A 67-year-old man arrived in the Emergency Admissions Unit with a painful, swollen big toe and has been unable to weight bear for the previous 2 days. On examination the toe is hot and erythematous, and tender to touch. He has a past history of peptic ulcer disease, for which he was admitted to hospital one year ago.

An X-ray demonstrates some soft tissue swelling but no bony fracture. A blood sample taken by the GP has shown a uric acid level of 16 mg/dL (normal range 3.5–7.2 mg/dL) and a normal white cell count. A joint aspiration in A&E has been sent to assess for birefringent crystals and microscopy and culture.

He is diagnosed with acute gout and you have been asked to write his prescription chart. He has no allergies.

CHART	PRESCRIPTION
Stat.	Indomethacin, 100 mg, p.o. Paracetamol, 1 g, p.o.
Regular	Indomethacin, 50 mg, p.o., q.d.s. Lansoprazole 30 mg, p.o., o.m. Paracetamol, 1 g, p.o., q.d.s. VTE prophylaxis as appropriate
P.R.N.	Morphine sulphate IR, 5 mg, i.v./p.o., Max 4-hourly Cyclizine, 50 mg, i.v./p.o., max t.d.s. Lactulose, 10 mL, p.o., max b.d. (for constipation)
Fluids	
CI/Stop	Stop all thiazides, angiotensin receptor antagonists and angiotensin converting enzyme inhibitors for 1/7 (review renal function). Stop other nephrotoxics including lithium, metformin, daptomycin, aminoglycosides. Stop aspirin.

If the patient is allergic to NSAIDs or has a history of a recent GI bleed, prescribe colchicine, 500 micrograms, p.o., q.d.s.

Continue allopurinol if patient is already on it for gout.

Do not add allopurinol until uric acid levels normalise and patient is well. Start allopurinol with either colchicine or NSAID cover, usually after 3–4 weeks, as it may precipitate a gouty attack.

Reference

Jordan KM, Cameron JS, Snaith M, *et al.* British Society for Rheumatology and British Health Professionals in Rheumatology guideline for the management of gout. *Rheumatology (Oxford).* 2007 Aug; **46**(8): 1372–4.

Endocrinology

17. Diabetic ketoacidosis

A 19-year-old female presents to A&E with abdominal pain and confusion. She has had Type 1 diabetes mellitus since childhood. Her friend informs you that last night she had attended a party and had forgotten to take her insulin. She has a GCS of 14/15 and ketotic fetor.

OBSERVATIONS	
Respiratory rate (breaths per minute)	26
Heart rate (beats per minute)	88
Blood pressure (mmHg)	119/72
Oxygen saturation (%)	98%
Temperature (°C)	37.0

Her blood results are as follows.

Glucose (mmol/L)	31
Na^+ (mmol/L)	142
K^+ (mmol/L)	5.9
Urea (mmol/L)	10.1
Creatinine (micromol/L)	128
eGFR (ml/min/1.73 m^2)	87
Blood ketones (mmol/L)	7.9

Arterial blood gas (on room air)

pH	7.19
PaO_2 (kPa)	14.1
$PaCO_2$ (kPa)	4.6
HCO_3^- (kPa)	13
Base excess	–7.1

You diagnose diabetic ketoacidosis on the basis of:

1. Acidosis (pH <7.3).
2. Hyperglycaemia.
3. Ketosis.

CHART	PRESCRIPTION
Stat.	Actrapid 50 units in 50 mL 0.9% saline at rate of 0.1 unit/kg/hr
Oxygen	2 L via nasal cannula, Target saturations 94–98% (PRN)
Regular	VTE prophylaxis as appropriate
P.R.N.	
Fluids	0.9% saline, 1 L, over 1st hour 0.9% saline, 1 L, 20 mmol KCL over next 2 hours 0.9% saline, 1 L, 20 mmol KCL over next 2 hours 0.9% saline, 1 L, 20 mmol KCL over next 4 hours 0.9% saline, 1 L, 20 mmol KCL over next 4 hours 0.9% saline, 1 L, 20 mmol KCL over next 6 hours
CI/Stop	

Two large-bore intravenous cannulae should be inserted for co-administration of sodium chloride and insulin.

An infusion of 50 units Actrapid in 50 mL of 0.9% normal saline should be started at a rate of 0.1 unit/kg/hr. The patient weighs 52 kg, so the infusion must be set at 5.2 units per hour or 5.2 mL per hour (as there are 50 units within a 50 mL infusion). *Six units per hour is started for the average adult.*

Re-evaluate the patient continuously. This involves hourly blood ketones, glucose and potassium (remember, insulin drives potassium into cells and leads to hypokalaemia).

Aim to reduce blood glucose concentrations by 5 mmol/L every hour. The rate of the infusion can be tailored to achieve this.

DKA has resolved when blood ketones <0.3 mmol/L and venous pH >7.3.

Once blood glucose <14 mmol/L, 10% dextrose can be used together with sodium chloride to prevent hypoglycaemia and augment fluid replacement. By this point, the patient should be ready to eat. Once DKA has resolved, the appropriate subcutaneous regime can begin.

The patient may require review by the diabetic specialist team if they have been newly diagnosed or require alteration of their normal insulin regime.

Reference

National Health Service Diabetes. *The Management of Diabetic Ketoacidosis in Adults*. NHS Diabetes; 2010.

18. Hypoglycaemia

A 29-year-old woman is an inpatient of the diabetic ward, having been admitted 4 days ago with diabetic ketoacidosis secondary to an episode of diarrhoea, which has since resolved. The nurse informs you that the patient has become increasingly confused, and that she is now very drowsy. On further questioning, you note that she has not been eating very much despite having started her normal insulin regime yesterday. The nurse informs you that her blood glucose is now 2.1.

You begin treatment for hypoglycaemia.

Treatment options:

- If conscious, Glucogel can be given orally.
- If unconscious, 20% dextrose, 75 mL, i.v. followed by a normal saline flush.
- If unconscious and no i.v. access, 1 mg, i.m. glucagon followed oral glucose when lucid.

CHART	PRESCRIPTION
Stat.	Glucogel, 1 tube, p.o.
Regular	Normal insulin regime (CROSS OFF NEXT DOSE AND DISCUSS TO REDUCE THE DOSE) VTE prophylaxis as appropriate
P.R.N.	Glucogel, 1 tube, p.o., and reassess BMs Glucagon, 1 mg, i.v./i.m., max o.d., reassess BMs
Fluids	
Caution	STOP Insulin and other antidiabetic drugs

Continuous reassessment of BMs, followed by assessment of current insulin regime. Ensure sugary drinks and meal after event.

Reference

Diabetes NHS. *The Hospital Management of Hypoglycaemia in Adults with Diabetes Mellitus*. NHS Diabetes; 2010.

Electrolyte abnormalities

19. Hypercalcaemia

A 58-year-old male is an inpatient of your ward. He has a background history of squamous cell carcinoma of the lung, which was recently found to have metastasised to bone. For the last few hours he has been vomiting and complaining of abdominal pain. You check his latest blood results and they are as follows.

Na^+ (mmol/L)	142
K^+ (mmol/L)	3.8
Urea (mmol/L)	6.7
Creatinine (micromol/L)	132
eGFR (mL/min/1.73 m^2)	78
Ca^{2+} (mmol/L)	3.2
Albumin	26
ALP	142
Inorganic PO^{4-}	1.15

On examination, his observations are stable, although he has dry mucous membranes. You make a diagnosis of hypercalcaemia, likely due to bony metastases, on the basis of:

1. Hypercalcaemia
2. Hypoalbuminaemia
3. Hyperphosphataemia
4. High ALP.

Write up a drug chart for the treatment of hypercalcaemia. You should aim for 1) fluid repletion and 2) limiting bone resorption using a bisphosphonate.

CHART	PRESCRIPTION
Stat.	
Oxygen	
Regular	VTE prophylaxis as appropriate
P.R.N.	
Fluids	0.9% saline, 300 mL + pamidronate 30 mg over 3 hours through a large vein AND 0.9% saline, I L, stat + 20 mmol KCL through a different vein 5% dextrose, I L, over 8 hr + 20 mmol KCL 5% dextrose, I L, over 8 hr + 20 mmol KCL
Caution	

20. Hyperkalaemia

You are on a general medical ward, nearing the end of your shift. You are checking blood results of patients on your ward, and you notice that a patient has a Potassium of 6.9 mmol/L. The patient is 41 years old and has recently been treated for a pneumonia. She is on day 4 of a 5-day course of co-amoxiclav, and has intravenous fluids running. She started eating and drinking this morning.

She appears clinically well but does complain of some light-headedness.

You request an ECG, which shows signs of hyperkalaemia (which may include the following: small/absent P waves, broad QRS complexes, tall tented T waves, AV conduction block, VF, sine wave rhythm).

You must stop any on-going intravenous infusions containing potassium. Protect the myocardium by prescribing calcium chloride, move extracellular potassium into the intracellular compartment and remove potassium from the body. Write a prescription chart as appropriate.

CHART	PRESCRIPTION
Stat.	10% calcium chloride, 10 mL, i.v. over 2 min Salbutamol, 20 mg, Neb
Oxygen	
Regular	Calcium resonium, 15 g, p.o./p.r., q.d.s. VTE prophylaxis as appropriate
P.R.N.	Salbutamol, 5 mg, Nebs, Max 4-hourly
Fluid	10 units Human Insulin in 500 mL 10% dextrose, over 15–30 minutes
CI/Caution	Do not add potassium to i.v. fluids Consider withholding ACE inhibitors, ARBs Stop any potassium sparing agents (e.g. spironolactone) Calcium chloride potentiates the effects of digoxin and can prompt digoxin toxicity

Reassess fluid balance and monitor BMs hourly.

N.B. 10 units Human Insulin is given in glucose 50 g i.v. (i.e. 500 mL of 10% dextrose or 250 mL of 20% dextrose).

Reference

University Hospitals of Leicester NHS Trust. *Guideline for the Management of Acute Hyperkalaemia in Adult Patients*. Acute Division, University Hospitals of Leicester NHS Trust; Sept 2011.

21. Hypernatraemia

A 68-year-old female patient is on an elderly care ward having been in hospital for 2 weeks. She was initially admitted having suffered a fall and suffered a Colles' fracture. Her rehabilitation was going well, and she was awaiting a social care package to be put into place prior to her return home.

You return to the ward on Monday, and have been told that the patient has developed a UTI, and has been declining food and drink over the weekend. She was prescribed i.v. antibiotics and fluids yesterday.

Currently, she is not oriented in time and place and scores 3/10 on the AMTS, having scored 9/10 the week before. She appears clinically dry.

You check her blood tests, which were sent yesterday:

Na^+ (mmol/L)	158
K^+ (mmol/L)	5.2
Urea (mmol/L)	10.1
Creatinine (micromol/L)	128
eGFR (mL/min/1.73 m^2)	87
WCC (10^9/L)	9.8
Hb (g/dL)	13.2
MCV (fL)	89

The weekend doctor had inserted a cannula, but the patient has removed this. The history and blood results demonstrate that the patient is dehydrated.

You reinsert a cannula, securing it using a bandage and prescribe:

1 L 0.9% saline over 4 hours
1 L 0.9% saline over 4 hours
1 L 5% dextrose + 20 mmol K^+ over 6 hours

You recheck the U&E later in the afternoon and prescribe i.v. fluids to correct her hypernatraemia. Note: other causes of hypernatraemia include primary hyperaldosteronism, diabetes insipidus and osmotic diuresis. In this scenario, the patient's history and high urea and creatinine signify dehydration.

N.B. Although 0.9% saline contains the entire sodium requirement per litre for 1 day's maintenance, this patient is clinically underfilled, and normal saline is relatively hypotonic in a 'hypertonic' patient.

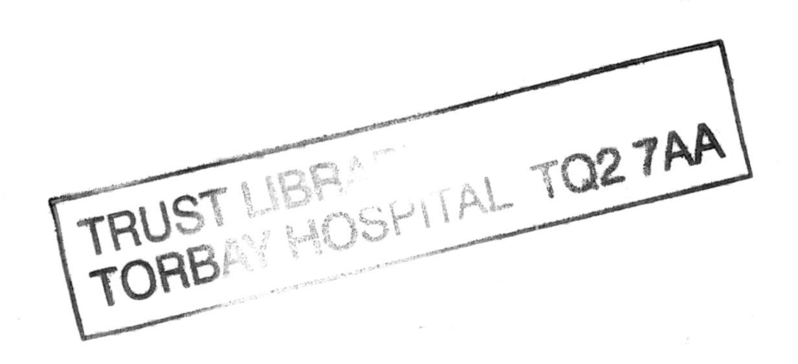

22. Anaphylaxis

A 39-year-old female was admitted to the Surgical Admissions Unit, with symptoms consistent with acute cholecystitis. She has a penicillin allergy. She was started on intravenous ceftriaxone.

Five minutes after her first dose, she develops a worsening rash across her extremities and a sudden onset wheeze. She complains of shortness of breath and a headache. On examination, she is pruritic and has evidence of peri-oral angioedema. Her observations are:

OBSERVATIONS	
Respiratory rate (breaths per minute)	35
Heart rate (beats per minute)	92
Blood pressure (mmHg)	102/52
Oxygen saturation (%)	93%
Temperature (°C)	37.2

This patient has signs and symptoms of an IgE-mediated hypersensitivity reaction, i.e. anaphylactic shock. She is likely to have had a reaction to ceftriaxone.

The patient is seriously unwell. You call for urgent senior help, approach the patient using an ABCDE approach, and stop the offending drug.

You then administer **15 L oxygen via non-rebreathing bag** and initiate treatment as follows:

- Adrenaline (1:1000) 500 micrograms i.m.
- 0.9% saline, 500 mL i.v. Stat.
- Chlorphenamine 10 mg i.m./i.v. Stat.
- Hydrocortisone 200 mg i.m./i.v. Stat (after initial resuscitation).

Adrenaline can be given again after 5 minutes if there is no clinical improvement. Monitor the airway closely and consider airway adjuncts (or contact on-call anaesthetist) if there is further concern.

The frequency of cephalosporin cross-reaction in a penicillin-allergic patient is approximately 10%. You document this allergy in the prescription chart and consult the hospital guidelines for an alternative antibiotic therapy.

After the acute management, remember to report the adverse reaction to the Medicines and Healthcare Products Regulatory Agency (MHRA) using the yellow card scheme (www.mhra.gov.uk).

At discharge, refer the patient to an allergy clinic to ascertain the exact cause.

Reference

Resuscitation Council. *Emergency Treatment of Anaphylactic Reactions*. Working Group of the Resuscitation Council (UK); 2008.

Index